The Good
& The Ugly

GROWING THE GOOD, BREAKING THE BAD
& UNDOING THE UGLY IN PARAMEDICINE

Tammie Bullard

Resounding Impact Publishing

PERTH | WESTERN AUSTRALIA

www.gbuparamedic.com

Book Layout ©2017 BookDesignTemplates.com

Ordering Information:

Quantity sales. Special discounts are available on quantity purchases by corporations, associations, and others. For details, contact the author via the website listed above.

The Good, The Bad & The Ugly Paramedic by Tammie Bullard 2nd ed.

ISBN 978-0-6488808-0-6

What a fabulous book! Honest, insightful and invaluable to all in this profession. I will be strongly recommending this great book to my students and the wider paramedic community. Really well done!

Lisa Holmes, Lecturer in Paramedicine, Edith Cowan University

What a thought-provoking book. I recognised a lot of the situations from my own experiences. This book has re-motivated me to strive for the best patient-centred care, and I have recently had more courage to challenge others' behaviour that prevents this.

Holly, Paramedic

The "we" tone of The Good, The Bad & The Ugly Paramedic allows the reader to feel like we're all in this together and working towards the same goal. Throughout reading, I could think of at least a dozen people I'd love to give the book to, myself included. This will be such a great resource for students and preceptors, really useful.

Anna, Paramedic Preceptor

This was a thoroughly enjoyable book that reminded me of myself at many stages throughout my career. It brought to mind that despite my best intentions to uphold a standard, there have been times where the bad the ugly have crept in. I am grateful to have been reminded of it. It would be a good book for junior paramedics to read as they reach the senior stage of their training, and then again every few years or so throughout their careers. I have been in this line of work for nearly thirty years and it brought a lot to mind for me to think about.

Trevor, Station Manager

For Joe & Alex

Your unwavering encouragement, constant support,
brave and open honesty, laughter and love
make the world a great place.

*"Life doesn't require that we be the best,
only that we try our best."*

—H JACKSON BROWN JR

CONTENTS

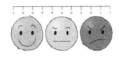

WHY THIS BOOK
& WHY IT MATTERS

Thank you for choosing to read this book, a work in progress for four years, finally on paper, much to my surprise after all this time!

It has been written specifically for paramedics, by a paramedic, but with the combined thoughts, words, ideas, tips and opinions of at least one thousand others.

I have tried counting the number I have worked alongside, learned from, trained with, taught, spoken to, listened to, observed or connected with throughout my career, that helped to form each chapter, but I can only estimate.

Something that I never have, and never will, claim to know, is what makes a good paramedic. Like everyone, I have my ideas around how that looks, but it's simply not my place to define this. Instead, it's up to each of us to identify what makes us feel like we're giving our best, and that will differ for everyone.

The good, bad and ugly sliding scale, used in this book, is designed to illustrate to us, as individuals, where we're at, just like the pain scale we use in our daily patient care. This way, we can visualise our habits, picture our behaviours and ascertain how good, bad, or ugly our paramedic practice may feel, on any given day.

As in many aspects of life, the moral dilemmas we face throughout a prehospital career, are often related to our behaviours. This means that we undoubtedly find ourselves on a continuous journey of self-reflection, in order to feel satisfied, successful and safe.

Away from the ambulance, even writing this book throws up the types of ethical quandary that can threaten those basic needs. What if someone gets annoyed about the bad habits highlighted? How will I feel if all of my colleagues disagree with what they read? Am I risking industry-wide scorn by putting these words on paper?

I almost ditched the entire project several times, but then, at the insistence of my family, I began to test the waters by talking about the book concept to some of my peers.

It was suddenly fascinating to hear comments that some are embarrassed by their behaviour, but the longer they leave it, the harder it becomes to make a change. Several described a desire to provide their absolute best to patients but brought to light the difficulties around maintaining this in the long term. Others mentioned bad habits that they've developed, or how their standards seem to have slipped, but outlined the more natural path of taking shortcuts.

To my horror, I also heard from some that they feel caught up in bad behaviours, because they have come to form part of their connection with groups of colleagues, or they have shaped their work persona around such attitudes, so it feels too late for change.

Hearing the open, honest and brave words from those paramedics, about their self-loathing, or their desire to wipe the slate clean with a fresh approach, makes it easy to maintain my conviction. New motivation to deliver a book that encourages all of us just to take a minute and reassess.

With questions such as "Why bother when so many others don't?" coming up in so many conversations, I decided that I'd rather face some negativity than ignore the potential to encourage positive change.

Like everyone else in this world, I am not perfect in any of my chosen roles, personally or professionally. I will never claim to know the best thing to do in any situation or have all of the answers. Some of the good, bad and ugly examples that follow, I confess that I have engaged in myself. What I have learned from these situations though, is that I always regret any bad or ugly action, or inaction immediately.

This regret has been known to keep me awake at night, particularly at the beginning of my career when I was keen to fit in and more frightened of going against others. It sometimes felt like I let down my patients, my colleagues and my family. When they trust me to do the right thing, simply because I say that I will, it's vital that I aim to meet those expectations that I have set, without fail.

I still catch myself occasionally now, in situations where I'm not proud of particular behaviours, but have learned over time that there's only one way to stop myself falling into repetitively bad habits. Continual self-reflection around everything I do, while I'm doing it, so there's no need to think about it once I head towards home.

I have also learned, unfortunately, how uncomfortable it can feel to speak up in challenging situations, rather than sweep them under the rug. This never gets easier but knowing that most other paramedics support and believe in best patient care, safety and overall professionalism, makes it worth stepping into that discomfort when necessary. With this in mind, encouraging readers of this book that they're not alone when the need arises to discuss challenges with their peers, may go some way towards providing that support.

All of the examples in the scenarios you're about to read have actually happened. I have either witnessed them in action, acted them out myself, or heard about them from others, so it's as realistic as it can be in written format. For this reason, I have refrained from quoting any specific situation, conversation, phrase, or story in its entirety.

If any reader feels that they recognise themselves somehow, they can rest assured that they are not alone. Also, no scenario included is a one-off example. The only inclusions are those that come up on multiple occasions, therefore rendering them worthy of discussion.

Before publishing, it has been a privilege to have such a kind and generous group of beta readers, willing to read and critique this book. Some new to prehospital care, some with decades of experience and some non-paramedics included. I am full of respect and admiration for each of them. Their honest, open, thoughtful approach, despite any discomfort, is the ultimate tool for me to improve, both my writing and my practice.

To every single paramedic I have encountered over the years, I am grateful for your part in shaping my career. I wish I could credit each person for their input, but there are just too many to mention.

For those who have spoken openly about work-related behaviours, shared stories of frustration and success, made positive changes and talked about the experience, mentored, tutored, educated, supported or challenged me, I am eternally grateful.

As a side note, on the day that this book was sent in draft format to the beta reading group, I found myself putting it all temporarily on hold. I got to observe healthcare behaviours *firsthand, as one of my sons was electrocuted and rendered unconscious.*

Although we've been through injury and illness in the past, it was the first time as a parent, and paramedic, that I found myself entirely dependent on the hope that he would be treated just as well as each caregiver's family members would wish for.

Despite the friendly, compassionate approach of some, the remainder left us frustrated, confused and dismayed. It was an extremely unpleasant eye-opener for me. Stark evidence of how much the demeanour, tone of voice, action and inaction of medical professionals impact upon those who trust in our care.

This account is not a resentful or vindictive addition to the book. I include it simply to highlight the words of my son when we came home. "I'd rather be electrocuted again, than ever feel as worthless and annoying as I have done over the past two days."

Poignant timing to make me more determined than ever to publish.

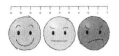

GUIDELINES FOR
THE GOOD, THE BAD
& THE UGLY

We love our guidelines, or we're familiar with them at least, so what better way to start than to set out a pattern to follow when reading this book? If you're like the majority of humans, you will have an inherent desire to do the right thing. If you genuinely are like most humans, however, you probably also have a similar wish to make life easier.

With this in mind, The Good, The Bad & The Ugly Paramedic is a friendly companion that supports you in finding your own, individual, healthy balance between the two.

From hereon in, throughout each chapter, unless it's a direct question or call to action, there will be no further reference to you, the individual. With a clear goal to help the reader self-reflect, without judgement, shame or accusation, taking the team-based "we" approach may help us to assess our moral compass more effectively.

Through conversational tone, reading this book should feel similar to that of paramedics chatting in an ambulance, or on station. A setting in which we feel safe to share our thoughts and see how we measure up to our own, and perhaps others' professional expectations.

It's not a textbook about skills or knowledge, not by a long shot! We read plenty of those to learn our craft, and no doubt continue to do so. Instead, this one is entirely attitude based upon how we choose to manage our professional careers. By highlighting examples of good, bad and ugly approaches through the scenarios we're about to read, it takes a similar approach to the hands-on training we're most familiar with, by putting us in the shoes of the paramedics involved. The aim of the game is that we can work towards:

Maintaining good, in fact, excellent, standards of patient care as a matter of course, rather than easing off over time.

Taking pride in standing our ground as individuals, sticking to what we believe in, rather than feeling pressured into joining a different crowd.

Inciting passion in new paramedics, and reigniting enjoyment in the role, for those who may have lost their initial spark.

Ensuring continuing attention to safety measures and safe practices, rather than cutting corners and increasing risk.

Enhancing public and interprofessional respect for prehospital care through our choices, rather than damaging reputations hard-earned over the decades.

Preventing unnecessary grievance or legal action from affecting our jobs, and professional registrations, rather than providing any reason for complaint.

Cutting out negative comments towards colleagues doing a good, thorough job, rather than encouraging any favourable inferences of being complacent.

Encouraging open, honest and transparent conversation to learn from each other, and our mistakes, rather than bluffing that "we've got this" in everything we do.

Establishing a community of good paramedics to support and encourage each other on road, in organisations and online, instead of seizing opportunities to criticise or mock.

Formulating consistent, reliable and replicable approaches to our practice so that it's just as acceptable for others, as it is for our families, rather than modifying standards to suit ourselves.

Checking in, from time to time, to reassess those standards, rather than remaining oblivious to changing behaviours until they're out of our control.

To reach these outcomes, the book itself takes a "pick up, put down, then pick back up again" approach. We can read a snippet when we're short on time or lose ourselves in the flow from start to finish. It's easy to skip forwards or backwards, without being concerned about missing connections in between, and each chapter summarises why each aspect matters, for a quick refresher whenever we need it.

Like a trusted colleague, who understands our role in-depth, we can come home to this book. Re-read highlighted areas that we resonate with and return to it whenever we want to reassess our practice, or our priorities, on the good, bad and ugly scale.

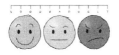

CHAPTER ONE

PUBLIC PERCEPTION
MEANS EVERYTHING

The fact that paramedics are in the public eye at such a high level is likely how we noticed the role in the first place. At some time in our lives, we may have experienced paramedic care ourselves. Perhaps we saw ambulances buzzing around the streets on lights and sirens. Or maybe we've watched television shows depicting the role in ways which have somehow caught our interest.

As none of us can be perfect all of the time, it's healthy to reflect on our performance within the public arena regularly throughout our careers. Are we heading in the right direction with our individual moral compasses? Are we happy with what we're putting out there?

The Good

Every single one of us starts our career hoping to be a fantastic paramedic, no matter how we choose to qualify that internally. Most of us are acutely aware and highly appreciative of the fact that we're in a position of immense public trust. Usually, we're keen to go out of our way to uphold this professional image, but there are times when it can be tempting to take shortcuts, particularly when we've been run ragged and are under pressure. Occasionally we may simply forget where we are, or who is around. We become so used to our role, and its environment, that any sense of feeling "at home" in a work setting, may begin to dull our professional senses.

There is a well-known expression that depicts this sneaky, difficult to notice, phenomenon perfectly. The situation in which we want our good paramedic scale to register off the charts, and we feel that it does. We go out of our way to do the right thing wherever possible. We aim for best patient care and the highest of high standards, but we may be letting ourselves down without even realising it. "Familiarity breeds contempt" as the saying goes. We become so familiar with certain aspects of our role that we begin to disregard things that could be, or perhaps should be, considered more often.

PLEASING THE PUBLIC -V- PROTECTING OUR PEACE

We've managed to snatch five minutes between jobs while our partner finishes paperwork. We're parked alongside the pavement outside a cafe, engine running, with a hot drink in hand. We've all experienced it, that sublime moment of the first taste of our coffee, or biting into a long-awaited sandwich and savouring the only chance we may get all day.

Just as we start to relax into it, a stranger walks up and knocks on the window to ask how they go about becoming a paramedic. We roll down the window and with a friendly smile, spend a minute or two telling them where to find further information. We wish them luck with their efforts, with an encouraging "Might see you on road in the future" type comment. It may not be the ideal accompaniment to our lunch. Still, we can quickly point them in the right direction, then look apologetic and explain that we must get our paperwork done at the same time as eating because there will be another job waiting as soon as we finish.

The unexpected visitor's trust and respect for paramedics not only remain intact, but the sandwich and coffee can continue without guilt or discomfort. Yes, it can be difficult to always be in full view of the public, especially during those brief snippets of downtime, but it's a highly visible position that we have chosen to hold. These encounters can make or break public perception if we handle it impolitely because we're tired and time-poor.

DELIBERATE DRIVING -V- CHAOS ON THE ROADS

As soon as our attending crew mate picks up the radio to notify control that we're available, we are dispatched on lights and sirens to a neighbouring suburb. We all know that emergency driving can be infuriating on busy roads. What is easy to forget, however, is that we, as paramedics, become entirely used to it, but it remains confusing and may often cause panic in regular road users.

With this in mind, we drive proactively. We aim to pick a lane and stick to it as much as possible, using indicator signals and educating other drivers to abide by the road rules through moving aside appropriately. We give those that have seen us approach, using their rear-view mirrors, time to predict which direction we're taking. We could perhaps get through the traffic quicker by zigzagging between vehicles and changing lanes repeatedly, but we know that this creates confusion and increases the chance of unnecessary accidents.

We use our beacons, flash our headlights and cycle through the various sirens, while ensuring that we leave enough distance between our vehicle and the drivers that haven't yet noticed us. We avoid rear-ending the driver who slams on the brakes when they suddenly realise we're behind them. We're also careful not to force drivers to enter an intersection, through a stoplight or sign, so that they don't risk being struck by other vehicles. When possible, we signal thanks to anyone helping to clear our path.

Growing legal liability on ambulance services naturally increases the pressure on response times but also results in higher numbers of priority calls. Public perception is of increased numbers of emergency ambulances, therefore how we behave on the roads is under more substantial scrutiny than ever before. Most of us have watched video footage of emergency vehicles struggling to get through traffic. We expect drivers on roads to let us pass safely, but how many of us have also watched the aggressive and erratic driving of some paramedics. Countless emergency service personnel have caused panic and stress amongst drivers en route to calls. If they have experienced such behaviours in the past, they may now be terrified, or even defensive, when we approach.

Our expectations of general road users can only match that of our own emergency driving. Otherwise, any double standards are unreasonable and unfair. Being confident and direct in the driving seat is necessary to forge safely ahead, but doing this courteously and professionally helps us to maintain a positive image, despite the need for urgency. Such an approach may ultimately keep our patients, other road users, ourselves and our crew mates safe, as well as our excellent reputations intact.

CLEANING UP OUR MESS -V- DESTROYING THE SCENE

Once we've reached our destination, we attend to an overdose at a bus stop and travel towards the emergency department with our now stable patient. While working at the roadside, we drop everything we discard into a rubbish bag and take it with us in the ambulance to dispose of later.

Many of us may notice on our days off, when we go out for a run, or walk the dog, discarded gloves and medical rubbish. We know it just has to be from an ambulance call. Leaving mess and chaos behind at a scene can damage our professional reputation in the public eye.

Even though dangerous environments, bad weather, darkness and urgency prevail, on most calls, good paramedics can still tidy up loose ends with minimal effort before transporting. We are not exempt from littering in our personal lives, so unless extreme circumstances prevail, we cannot assume to be exempt in uniform. Forming the habit of using a disposable bag, on every call, immediately cuts down the need to even consider this, we simply discard everything into it as we work. (With the additional benefit of creating an organised working space, it may also help us to avoid confusion in searching for items and reduce stress on scene.)

Whether in a patient's home or out on the street, if we throw everything we dispose of onto the floor as we work, somebody, at some point, has to clean it up. Dropping plastic squares from electrodes onto the floor, bed or couch in an older person's home during a twelve lead ECG seems innocuous. It leaves them with an invisible slip hazard later on, however, but only takes us a second to drop into a waste container. If we work on a dual response call, particularly with a cardiac arrest, there is usually at least one crew member left behind to drive the follow-up vehicle, when the patient is transported under priority conditions. Taking a couple of minutes to dispose of debris from the scene may reduce the psychological trauma experienced by family members or bystanders after the event.

Imagine a loved one is close to death and whisked away in an ambulance, then family members arrive home. We probably don't want them to see the discarded mess at the scene as a reminder of their pain, before having to collect it up and dispose of it.

Public perception of our professionalism and care extends so much further than clinical interventions. As a good paramedic, we can take many extra, small measures to ensure that our attention is appreciated, and the trust that we are privileged to feel remains protected in the long term.

The Bad

Most of us generally want to do the right thing, but sometimes it's easy to fall into bad habits, get caught up in what we see others get away with or succumb to pressure from colleagues who choose to discourage our positive behaviours.

PROFESSIONAL CHATTER -V- GOSSIPING GROUPS

No matter where we work in the world, most paramedics are accustomed to "ramping" or waiting in corridors and triage areas, with patients. In many countries, this wait may be several hours with each patient we transport, and results in extremely long periods, therefore, of public scrutiny. While some of us may view this waiting period as a form of relief from attending to continuous call outs, equally, some of us may detest the time spent awaiting a bed for our patient. Either way, it is becoming a growing part of our role and doesn't look like it will disappear any time soon.

So, we're standing in the corridor for long periods, what a great opportunity to catch up and have a chat with colleagues! We're talking about jobs we've done lately. Perhaps it's the fascinating but gruesome details of a murder-suicide or the humorously inappropriate behaviour of an intoxicated patient. Maybe we're discussing our frustrations around a regular caller whom we've now attended twice already this shift, or relaying the details of our alcohol-fuelled personal shenanigans during days off.

Imagine how our patient, and any family members they have with them, may perceive this? The longer they listen and observe our behaviour, the more damaging to our reputations this may be.

The best-case scenario for our professional reputation is that they lose respect for what they had previously considered an admirable career. The worst-case scenario is that the patient, or their escort, is shocked enough to either lodge a complaint or worry that they may be our next topic of hilarity and scorn.

Such thoughts will undoubtedly return to the patient the next time they consider calling an ambulance. None of us embarked on this career to cause discomfort or angst, so it's well worth avoiding for both professionalism and job satisfaction.

PROMOTING PARAMEDICINE -V- INJURING OUR IMAGE

After several hours of waiting, we're surprised by an unexpected opportunity to take a short break, as there are no outstanding calls (*I hear you laughing at that unlikely story!*). We're parked up near the beach with a much-needed coffee, chatting to our partner, with our feet up on the dashboard. The windows are open to catch that beautiful ocean breeze, and we're playing a favourite song a little louder than usual so that we can grab that feeling of pseudo freedom we desperately crave.

The little children walking past with their kindergarten teacher suddenly lose their own happy, innocent sense of freedom, once they get near to our vehicle. They were initially excited to see the ambulance from further away, and their eyes lit up at the teacher's suggestion to wander over for a visit. The closer they get, however, the more intimidated they start to feel by the noise and demeanour of our crew. Most of us love the adoration children have for our roles and our vehicles, but as we slip into bad habits, it's easy to forget how we may be perceived.

On our first day at work in an ambulance, we wouldn't have dreamed of lounging in the seat with our boots up on the dashboard in public. No way would we have cranked the stereo with the windows open from the new office that once made us so proud.

Remember that feeling of walking past intimidating teenagers when we were little? That's the last feeling we want to elicit in anyone around us. We signed up to instil public confidence in us during times of emergency and care for people who call for an ambulance.

There are often opportunities where we can listen to great music and even elevate our feet by resting them up on the dash (as long as we wipe it down afterwards of course).

Still, those opportunities must be limited to the times that we're parked up away from the public eye.

HUMBLE PROTESTATION -V- DISRESPECTFUL DIATRIBE

Our next call comes across the radio, to an elderly lady with chest pain. Once we reach our destination, the patient's daughter has already arrived and calmed her mother. This gives us plenty of time to build rapport and reassure our patient during assessment, treatment and preparation for transport.

During their general chatter with our attending partner while we're driving, en route to hospital, we hear the patient praising the hard work of paramedics and expressing her thanks for the "tireless efforts" she describes. It feels good to be appreciated, doesn't it? Our partner, however, responds with "it's just a job" and dismisses her thanks. Going on to describe a lazy profession who get to lounge around and sleep between calls.

The patient cannot believe this and hopes that her gratitude is only dismissed due to modesty and humility. She wants, and possibly needs, to think that her perception of paramedics as professional, hardworking, caring members of society is correct. If this is not the case, how can she feel confident that we want to provide that professionalism and care?

Her daughter joins in to describe the cheery and reassuringly calm manner of paramedics during their treatment of her mother in the past. Our partner, however, is keen to emphasise their casual, cool demeanour. They go on to quote "You call, we haul!" type phrases, stating that we only work for half of the year. They are omitting the fact that a good chunk of that time is spent working long shifts or sleeping to catch up afterwards. As we listen, we cringe with shame.

Public perception of our role is generally extremely positive. Simply acknowledging this positive praise with polite thanks can help patients to maintain their sense of safety, security and confidence in the service that we provide. Educating any misconception is useful, when necessary if managed appropriately. Conversely, shutting down positive feedback and describing an entire profession in such negative terms is unfair to patients, to our colleagues and our entire industry.

If we wish to describe ourselves personally as lazy, slack, or any other negative term, that's entirely up to the individual. We can easily convince the general public of this with our words, body language and attitude, without even realising it. In doing this, however, we may irreparably damage the hard-earned reputation and respect that paramedics have gained over one hundred years.

The Ugly

We may have forgotten most of our reasons for becoming a paramedic because we're tired and it's been a long, long time in the making. We may be suffering from stressors that make it difficult even to want to do the right thing. We may be new to the role and think that we will fit in better if we can portray a relaxed and casual attitude. We may have been drawn to paramedicine purely for its image so that self-image is our focus.

Whatever the reason, sometimes paramedics, just like all other professions, can behave in ugly ways without even realising it.

DRIVING OUR TEAM -V- DITCHING OUR DUTIES

It's our turn to drive, so, while transporting a patient to the emergency department, we put in our headphones and make a phone call to a friend or colleague throughout the entire journey.

Meanwhile, our partner is in the back of the ambulance, attending to the patient. They can both hear the conversation, and they both know that they're in the hands of an inattentive driver as well as an inattentive clinician.

Throughout treatment, we can't hear our partner calling out updates regarding vitals assessed or medications given; therefore, we're not working as part of that team other than in a driving capacity. If our partner receives a complaint regarding an accusation of mistreatment, errors in medication, inappropriate behaviour, or if their safety is compromised, we can't confirm or deny any part of that, as we are not fully aware of any aspect.

Should the patient have a complicated presentation, we cannot support our crew mate in making decisions regarding clinical care, if they need to discuss the case en route or afterwards. Most importantly, we are driving distracted with a colleague and patient in the vehicle. In some jurisdictions, this may be illegal. In others, it may be considered enough of a distraction to warrant prosecution in the event of an accident.

Did we ever imagine, when we submitted our initial job application, that we would choose to be the type of paramedic to wear headphones and completely switch off from their partner and patient care? We can almost guarantee that the patient will be quick to share their disappointment and loss of respect for paramedics with family members, friends, hospital staff and potentially, our managers or governing registration bodies.

APPRECIATING PRIVILEGE -V- INFLATING IMPORTANCE

Back to the good old food break example, and we find ourselves between calls once again. It's now almost dark, and we're hungry, so we decide to sit in, rather than eat takeaway in the ambulance for a change.

We park in a nearby disability spot, lock the vehicle, and, as we're walking towards the restaurant, we notice passers-by watching, in that naturally curious way that occurs whenever an ambulance pulls up. As we enter, we're unaware of the distaste on the faces of those who have noticed that we're about to get comfortable. Public perception drops to an all-time low. Not only have we taken one of the only parking spaces available for patrons with mobility issues, but we are doing so purely for our own needs, and it's not appreciated at all.

Doing so may cause a massive loss of respect and is potentially damaging for the next time we have no choice but to park awkwardly at a life-threatening emergency call. Social media often depicts images and video footage of public hostility. Occasionally including aggressive acts towards ambulances blocking parked cars, or traffic attendants who refuse to back down on issuing a ticket.

As a profession, we become frustrated and confronted by such behaviour. Still, it begs the question of how thoughtful decisions are when parking an ambulance or response car purely for personal needs. Yes, paramedics have to eat, but there are ways around this. We can park nearby, if possible, and walk just a little further. Should the closest available space be far enough to affect response times, we may have the option of one crew member staying with the vehicle.

If we make ugly or thoughtless choices, however, we can guarantee that they will be noticed, and they will ultimately affect public perception. How can we expect members of the public to differentiate between this, and actual necessity, during access and egress for emergency calls?

MAINTAINING SAFE DISTANCE VS AN UGLY APPROACH

Once we've eaten, it's still early on a Saturday night in the city, and we attend our third unconscious and potentially intoxicated patient for the shift. We're getting tired, it's cold, and the pavements bustle with noisy partygoers. As we step out of the ambulance, we walk over to the patient on the ground, lying face down, with hands comfortably forming a pillow under their head. They are snoring gently and smell strongly of alcohol.

Before our partner does anything else, they nudge the patient with the toe of their boot, so that they don't have to lean over and risk the patient striking out violently. In the eyes of the general public, this will likely appear to be the utmost level of unacceptable behaviour from a paramedic. While the training we have in safely approaching a patient may be minimal in many ambulance services, we all know of tried and tested ways in which we can approach the situation with professionalism, as well as caution.

The patient may be alcohol or drug-affected and may indeed have the potential to be violent. We must ask ourselves, however, whether we would find our chosen methods of assessing this type of call, acceptable to watch if it were our family member on the ground.

Imagine the description of this one small act circulating amongst the friends and family of every bystander at the scene. Furthermore, nowadays, it is safe to assume that many of our public interactions are captured in video on a smartphone. While this is annoying, frustrating and can feel invasive, it's a realistic reminder for each of us to align our practice with the reasons that inspired us to become a paramedic in the first place.

At the end of the day, the media gives the public what the public wants to see. They have a service to provide and naturally must feed demand. If we don't destroy prehospital public perception, we won't find many members of the public ready to jump aboard a negative media bandwagon. Instead, an automatic jump to our defense may continue to remain the norm.

Why It Matters

Keeping the general public on side is vital to every one of us for the duration of our careers. We're generally renowned for being trusted. In some countries, the people we care for have even voted us the most trusted profession, time and time again, but we need to remember that we rely on the same level of care in return.

If the subject of working conditions and fatigue for paramedics comes up in the media, we don't want the general public to dismiss our needs because we've convinced them that we're lazy and have an easy time of it. We need them to understand and empathise so that they care enough to vote in our favour.

When we head into a coffee shop or lunch bar to grab something on the run between calls, we appreciate, and often desperately hope that a stranger in the queue offers to let us jump ahead. Their kindness helps to ensure that we don't miss a brief opportunity to find sustenance on the run.

When it's dark and wet on the roads, our lives depend on every driver slowing down and giving us a wide berth, keeping us safe, and setting an excellent example to other, less considerate, road users passing by. Why would they bother if we give them no reason to care?

Every single time we walk through the door of a patient's home, we hope that the occupants have no intention of causing us harm. We absolutely must, therefore, uphold the great trust that the majority of patients and bystanders bestow upon us. If we don't, it would be dangerously arrogant to continue to expect such a warm welcome across every threshold.

On those awful occasions where we find ourselves under threat or facing direct violence, we depend on the public outrage that comes as a result of being trusted and respected in an increasingly dangerous role. Whether it's in the form of a bystander stepping in to face danger with us at their own risk, or whether it's advocating across social media platforms to drive judicial reform in favour of our safety. We depend on society as a whole to continue to care about paramedics, just as much as they expect us to care about them.

At different points in our careers, we hear talk of how public perception has changed. There are conversations about why the media portray paramedics poorly. We may chat with colleagues regarding our frustration around negative attitudes towards us increasing. What we must ask is why there seems to be a shift in perspective.

Do we notice ourselves, and our colleagues, behaving in ways that may surprise or shock the general public? Is our profession demanding respect, but forgetting that it's a mutual, two-way street? Could it be possible that attention-grabbing apparel, declaring our paramedic, superhero-style status on days off, when we're out of uniform, may suggest a sense of elitism? Are we part of the growing wave of self-glorification on social media, inviting inevitable public scorn for our arrogance?

Realistically, without downplaying the great work we do, we are paid to provide a service. If we begin to view ourselves as heroes, we risk expecting the rest of the world to treat us as such, and that may lead to bad, or ugly, entitled behaviour that knocks us off our pedestals at high speed.

In simple terms, people talk. If we damage one person's perception of our profession today, it's likely to become an interesting discussion when they arrive at work or home. The people that they then talk to are disappointed and possibly surprised, so they later talk to their colleagues or family too.

By the time that one person, we shocked, upset or disappointed moves on to a different topic, the ripple effect of that one event may have destroyed our profession's reputation entirely, or at least put it into question. This answer to such a problem may depend upon the attitude of the next paramedic they encounter. How will our behaviour shape their opinion in future?

Put Yourself In The Picture

Remember when you decided to apply for your first paramedic role? Do you recall desperately hoping that you would be selected from amongst the ridiculously high number of applicants you were up against?

What was your perception of paramedics at that early stage? No doubt you were full of admiration and respect for the profession, and hopefully still are.

With this in mind, we have to uphold and maintain that reputation every single day, without fail. For the benefit of our industry, our colleagues and ourselves.

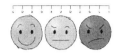

CHAPTER TWO

SAFETY DOESN'T HAVE
TO BE A DIRTY WORD

No matter which country, state, city or region we work in throughout the world, paramedic safety is a basic premise that we train to focus on intently, without fail. It's no accident that it forms the very first step of every primary survey before we even begin to think about our patient. It features heavily in every conversation during training, right through from assessing for potential danger upon entering a scene, to lifting and carrying appropriately. It's vital in keeping our patients, colleagues, bystanders, other emergency services and health professionals safe, as well as ourselves, so the reasoning behind such focus is perfectly understandable.

How many of us give this aspect of our work the level of focus it truly requires, however? Are we in the habit of using safety equipment and training to our best ability or do we learn to laugh in the face of such rules because we prefer to be seen as the mavericks of healthcare? Does peer pressure teach us to associate attention to safety with a "newbie" status, and we'd rather avoid risking the ridicule of our peers?

The Good

When we first began training, there is no doubt that almost every single one of us paid great attention to what we initially learned regarding safety. Most of us may recall thinking just how much we'd hate to be threatened or assaulted on the job and would do whatever it took to avoid the possibility of this happening. Many may have been fiercely passionate about avoiding risks in lifting, or using equipment appropriately so that we wouldn't have to face debilitating injury or health scares that may threaten our very livelihood. How high a priority does this remain for us, once we've notched up a year or two of service?

SAFETY FILLED -V- ADRENALINE FUELLED

On a Saturday night shift, we're dispatched to a paediatric cardiac arrest call as soon as we've logged in to our vehicle, and we're off and running right away. We know our partner well, and they are familiar with how we work, so there's no anxiety about the unknown or any unnecessary stress en route. We can feel safe to concentrate on our notebooks, calculating aloud drug doses appropriate for the patient's age, so that we can jot them down and ensure that we are as prepared as possible for the call.

As we pull up, our partner mentions that they will take an extra minute to reverse into the driveway so that it's quicker to retrieve and then load the stretcher, saving us several minutes on scene. We nod in agreement, feeling relieved to be starting a busy night shift with this type of partner. Confident enough to verbalise their thoughts, purely so that we are both on the same page, without seeking approval or comment. It's a great start.

The call goes as expected, CPR in progress as we extricate on the stretcher, into the ambulance, with the assistance of a backup crew, who arrive shortly after us. There's a lot to be done in the back of the ambulance en route; therefore, we need another paramedic to accompany us, so we weigh up the options. We know that our crew mate is an excellent, safe driver who does a great job of not getting distracted by the adrenaline rush of a paediatric resuscitation call and excels in commentary emergency driving. As much as we'd love to use their clinical assistance, we opt to have them transport us.

We choose this option despite an offer from one of the backup paramedics proudly declaring they'd "have us there in no time." We have noticed in the past that they like to speed through intersections and fly around corners without warning.

En route, we appreciate the decision as our crew mate calls out clear warnings of left or right turns and notifies us of upcoming braking and sudden changes that may affect our footing. We notice them scanning the windscreen, windows, mirrors and blind spots as they traverse busy roads while flicking their eyes to the rear-view mirror, maintaining awareness of either paramedic standing up.

Before clinical interventions, we let them know what's about to happen so that they call out on reaching a smooth patch of road. Or they slow down enough to aid efforts in safely carrying out more intricate skills. Our primary survey and status updates, called aloud for the benefit of all crew members, including the driver, are met with calm and attentive acknowledgment from the front seat.

With no need for excessive speed, the entire group is transported safely, pre-empting traffic as far ahead as possible to avoid becoming blocked in and having to stop. Still maintaining excellent control, they provide precise warning of our impending arrival, giving a chance for equipment to be gathered in the back of the ambulance, for rapid movement from the vehicle to the resuscitation bay.

As soon as we arrive, they step out quickly, in time to prevent adrenaline-fuelled helpers pulling the trolley out prematurely, avoiding stretcher collapse, potential injuries, dislodgement of airway adjuncts or IV lines, and unnecessary stressors in general. We wheel the patient into the emergency department and, while our partner assists the receiving team in transferring the patient, they maintain calm but firm control over the hands now rushing to remove ambulance equipment. They free us up to gather our thoughts so that we can provide a clear handover.

It all sounds a bit dreamlike, doesn't it? It doesn't seem stressful enough to depict an actual paediatric cardiac arrest call. It doesn't have to though.

We have all probably, hopefully, worked at least one shift, roster or rotation with a partner who makes things run smoothly. We feel safe with them. Life feels good. When we have a partner of this calibre, we find ourselves in that fortunate situation whereby no amount of our job-related focus is spent on their side of operations.

If we can be that driver, if we can provide our attending partner's brain with the freedom to concentrate on excellent clinical care, especially on high acuity calls, we participate equally in ultimately providing best patient care.

RESPECTING GUT FEELING -V- IGNORING INSTINCT

Once we've had a quick cup of coffee and debriefed with our colleagues from the backup crew, we clean up, restock and complete our paperwork before heading out towards a respiratory call for a patient who has asthma.

We pull up outside a house that appears to be in total darkness and, as we step out of the ambulance and reach for our equipment, our partner states that they have a sick feeling in the pit of their stomach.

We stop for a second and look at them directly, so that they know we're actively listening, and ask why they feel uncomfortable, only to find that they can't identify it, there just seems to be something "off" about the scene. We're well aware that there is potential for our patient to be deteriorating towards respiratory arrest inside the house. Still, in good paramedic style, we reach a compromise rather than mock or ignore our colleague's gut instinct.

The fact that no-one is waiting at the door, and that there are no lights on, could be suspicious, or it could just mean that the patient is in bed, in darkness, home alone. Either way, the fact that we'd expect our partner to respect our gut instinct means that we must also respect theirs.

As we're about to dial control to obtain more details from the original call taker, the phone rings with an urgent warning not to enter the scene. We jump back into the ambulance, and our partner drives off quickly as the story unfolds regarding a hoax caller who has been hiding in the darkness, in empty homes, intending to steal drugs from responding paramedics as they arrive.

The call taker picked up on some minor peculiarities and also identified with something "not sounding quite right" about this call, therefore notified their manager who ultimately confirmed our partner's suspicion.

Now, it may not always be as dramatic as that. It may be as simple as the suggestion of a different way to extricate a patient or having concerns about using a particular medication. As we all know, though, there exists an extremely fine line in this area.

If our partner ordinarily refrains from interfering, or playing standover tactics, and does not try to discredit us, or make us look foolish in front of others, we are more likely to respect them. If they stop themselves from interrupting unnecessarily to ask questions of our patient, support our treatment decisions and generally work with us in favour of best patient care, when they do suddenly choose to voice an opinion, it's probably worth listening.

Their gut instinct or specific knowledge in some area may save us our job. It may save our patient from disaster. It may only save us a little time and a little muscle effort, but more importantly, it may save our lives.

If we expect others to listen to our concerns and gut instincts, we absolutely must afford the same respect to our colleagues. If they are constantly interfering, butting in or undermining us though, they'll soon find that they have to speak an awful lot louder when they do have a real concern. For the good paramedic's part in it, encouraging crew mates to speak up is the reputation we're aiming for. Our patients, our personal lives and our professional careers depend on it.

STANDING FIRM -V- SEEKING EASY SOLUTIONS

It's now that awful time of the night shift, around three o'clock in the morning, and we're both tired. It feels like all of our equipment gets heavier as time goes on, and it's a struggle to feel enthusiastic about anything at this stage. We arrive at a nursing home and are ushered in quietly, towards an elderly patient. She sits on the edge of her bed, next to her husband, with several bags at her feet. Our patient feels anxious and has asked the nursing home staff to call for an ambulance so that she can be assessed in hospital.

We know that it's not an ideal place to be in the early hours of a weekend morning. We know community-based options would best serve our patient, but we also know that the nursing home cannot refuse the patient's request. Her husband cannot drive her there, and in many jurisdictions, ambulance transport cannot be refused if the patient wishes to attend the ED.

We ascertain that the patient's vitals are within appropriate parameters and begin walking her to the ambulance. Upon entering the vehicle, the patient demands that her husband travels with her, sitting together on the edge of the stretcher.

We gently explain that this is not possible. We offer the options of sitting up in a seat or lying on the stretcher, her husband seated nearby, still within reach to hold her hand. She refuses outright and just will not budge on this.

Both crew members look at each other, knowing that this is the worst time of night to require such a difficult negotiation. The glance we exchange also reassures us both, however, that we are not transporting without safety belts in place, just because we're tired, in the hope of making the job easier.

We explain to the patient once again, more firmly now, that there are no more options. We understand that she wishes to remain next to her husband for comfort, and we have provided an opportunity to satisfy that requirement, but sitting next to each other on the bed will not be happening.

The conversation continues for another fifteen minutes. We attempt to seek assistance from the patient's husband, but he can't persuade her either. We step outside and discuss potential options with our partner and ascertain, together, that there is no justification in calling for police backup or using chemical sedation. We simply need to maintain a united front and keep reiterating the same information.

Eventually, our patient tires of the conversation and lays down on the stretcher, upset and frustrated by the situation, but lying on the bed, nonetheless. We seize the opportunity to murmur our thanks, along with reassurances by way of distraction, as we gently secure the safety belts and cover them up with warm blankets for comfort.

Our partner quietly gestures to the elderly husband to fasten his seatbelt, in the seat closest to the stretcher, before safely stowing the patient's luggage and closing the doors, ready to commence transport.

There are countless ways for us to take almost undetectable shortcuts in terms of using safety equipment, restraints, straps and belts, as well as justify our decisions. We may suggest that a need for rapid transport means there is no time to fix the paediatric harness to the stretcher, so we transport the toddler in an ill-fitting adult harness instead.

We know that the safety belts can interfere with a twelve lead ECG, so we decide to leave them off, even though we could easily replace them once the reading is acquired. Perhaps we feel that a child is crying too much to place on the stretcher as they will only stop when we let a parent hold them. Maybe it means less lifting if we leave monitoring equipment on the back of the bed during transport, rather than moving it to a secure location then replacing it on arrival.

In a small number of cases, there will indeed be a clear justification in not using specified equipment. In most situations, however, no matter how we choose to explain or justify our decision, the pivotal moment will be when something goes wrong. We will more than likely be full of remorse for not having used the available safety equipment.

Every paramedic in the vicinity will want to give us their opinion about what we should have done, or could have done, or what they would have done. Our employer or professional governing body may find our decision not to use provided safety apparatus inexcusable, so we may lose our jobs, or at least be reprimanded. A patient, family member or injured partner may take legal or civil action against our decision. Even worse, severe injury or death may occur in a situation that could have been prevented.

If we find ourselves reluctant to bother with safety equipment, a quick thought towards the worst-case scenario outcome will generally provide the type of painful visual required, informing our best course of action.

Ultimately, the less we have to justify inaction around utilising government legislated, or ambulance service specified, safety equipment, the more comfortable and safe our lives and careers naturally become.

The Bad

As much as we may loathe the bad habits that we notice in others, can we honestly say that we are entirely faultless, every single day, without fail? It's unlikely.

Often, it's highlighted most clearly to us when we notice ourselves putting colleagues in situations that cause them to question our behaviour.

MAINTAINING SAFE MEASURES -V- CHANCING OUR LUCK

We decide to do an overtime shift with a paramedic we've never worked with before. Their reputation suggests that they're fun to work with and colleagues tell us in advance that we'll "have a blast" with this person, so we're looking forward to making some extra money in what sounds like a pleasant environment. After the first half an hour preparing the ambulance and equipment, we realise for ourselves that this person is bright, breezy, hilarious and the mood is set for a fantastic shift.

On the way to our first call, we dig out our stethoscope, safety glasses and pen torch while chatting, at which our partner laughs loudly from the driving seat, asking "What are you, a rookie?" They tell us "Relax, it's only a medical call, you won't need your glasses."

We begin to respond that we always take them into calls but then get frustrated at the need to justify ourselves, so just laugh it off along with them and soon arrive at the patient's home. A little embarrassed about the whole conversation and keen to return to the easy-going, fun mood we were enjoying earlier, we break from our regular routine and leave the glasses behind to avoid further mocking.

Our patient is vomiting blood, and immediately we regret that decision but continue without much choice. We ask our partner to draw up an intramuscular antiemetic in the hope that it starts working before we gain IV access. We notice that our partner is already administering the medication, while we're checking the patient's vitals, and feel a sense of dread when they place the used needle on top of our drug bag as we realise that things are beginning to feel a little unsafe.

Rather than create tension or discredit our partner in front of the patient, we ask if they can prepare the stretcher outside the front door. As soon as they leave, we discreetly pop the discarded needle into the sharps container, dig out a pair of work issue safety glasses from the base of the treatment bag, then check the name and expiry on the empty ampoule to ensure that the unchecked drug was correct. A quiet sigh of relief escapes our lips as we get back on track and attempt to regain control of the situation to avoid anything going unnecessarily wrong.

Our partner groans and begins to laugh when they re-enter the house and see that we've donned safety glasses, making jokes to the patient about some paramedics being "sticklers for the rules." We don't care at this point. We realise that we're working with a paramedic who would rather be complacent with safety, but in doing so, is risking the safety of patients and colleagues purely out of choice. This doesn't necessarily make them a bad paramedic, but it's bad practice and unfair to others.

With this single job alone, we now find ourselves having to spend extra time and attention on looking out for what our partner is doing, or not doing, just to maintain safety, throughout the rest of the shift. We're not precepting an intern, this is an experienced paramedic, so it's a frustrating and disappointing situation.

While nothing has gone wrong, we've already been at risk of blood and vomit contamination, a needlestick injury, and a drug error. Purely because our partner takes more pride in demonstrating their fun and easy-going persona, than adhering to the simple rules of basic safety that we have all been taught. Suddenly, the rest of the shift doesn't feel like it's going to be that much fun after all.

ENSURING ESCAPE -V- STRANDED & SCARED

After a few more calls, we've settled in and have established a routine of ignoring jibes about our need to "do the right thing," and we're relieved to notice that our partner has given up with most of the jokes because we're not rising to the bait. Thankfully, we haven't had to have any problematic conversations as nothing has gone irreparably wrong, so everyone is relatively happy.

En route to a head injury call at a local bar, we chat about upcoming days off and look forward to the plans we've made outside of work. We step out of the ambulance and begin walking into the scene, checking that our partner has their radio. They nonchalantly tell us that they never take it, laughing that we carry ours like a newbie, but they don't see the point as it's better to fly under the dispatch radar.

Our sense of foreboding is back, but we've just walked through the door and bystanders are already beckoning as the crowd swamps us.

The caller hadn't mentioned that this was a brawl and that there were several patrons still fighting. The only information given to the call taker was that someone was injured. As we're about to hit the duress button, our partner snatches the radio from us, so that they can converse with control to request urgent assistance, and we attempt to push our way back towards the exit.

Thankfully, some of the customers and security staff have noticed and do their best to chaperone us out safely, away from the fighting and aggressive, drunken demands to attend to the injured. We make a run for it back to the ambulance. At this stage, we're livid!

As our partner drives out of the car park to escape the mounting aggression, we take a couple of deep breaths to avoid venting too furiously and ask what they were thinking. Why did they grab the radio and leave us with no means of communication when they had earlier mocked our decision to carry it? Thankfully, we immediately notice their remorse.

While we settle and await police response around the corner, they mention their reluctance to be ridiculed. Talking about purposely not taking a radio or phone because some peers not only discourage it but blatantly mock them. They've watched others be teased for looking like a probationer, and have heard some boast that if dispatch can't contact them, they get to pick and choose when they respond to calls.

As with most examples throughout this book, it has to be assumed that no paramedic, at least we hope not, sets out to behave badly and certainly does not intend to cause harm due to action or inaction. Through forgetfulness, fear of ridicule, complacency or arrogance, some of us may see our radios, phones and occasionally, even our ambulance keys as less critical over time. How can that be so?

The harsh reality is that the moment we step away from the ambulance, car, pushbike, motorbike, van, bus, helicopter, aeroplane or whatever mode of transport we use, we are immediately vulnerable.

Without the safety of a vehicle, we cannot escape in any way other than running. How easy is that in a restrictive uniform and safety boots, relying solely on our level of fitness and speed?

With no means of communicating with control, we have absolutely no way to ask for assistance. We become stranded at the mercy of whatever situation we find ourselves in.

Without a radio or phone, for contacting each other, if disaster strikes when one of us is treating the patient, and the other is collecting the stretcher from the ambulance, we are completely alone and at extreme risk.

Similarly, unless both crew members carry a set of keys, one may be unable to re-enter the ambulance, should we be under threat, need to seek shelter, escape or make an urgent request for backup.

It may be evident to most, but it may take a near-miss for others to understand that our most essential items of kit absolutely must be our means of communication, and our means of escape.

PHYSICAL PROTECTION -V- INVINCIBLE RISK

Finally, we're on our last job of what's turned out to be an exhausting day. We can't wait for it to be over, although thankfully, we notice that our partner has now stopped making jokes about how they perceive our safe practices.

We're on our way to what sounds like a simple fall, for an assisted lift, before we head home.

When we arrive, we see that our bariatric patient is propped up against the wall, sitting on a carpeted surface, smiling and stating that they're uninjured, but requesting assistance to get up from the floor. The patient mentions that this isn't the first time this has happened, and previous ambulance crews have called for help with a lifting device.

We could hear en route that the radio is incredibly busy and just know that it's going to take forever for a low acuity backup response to reach us. So we carry on with our assessment and rule out obvious potential injury or medical cause for the fall within ten minutes of arriving.

At this point, we've decided in our mind that we'll be able to help the patient get to their feet without having to wait for backup. We go to the gym every day, we're exceptionally fit and strong, and there's no way we want to hang around for hours, we're already late finishing the shift as it is. We turn to our partner and ask them to grab a bed sheet or lifting belts from the ambulance, so we can utilise them in assisting our patient to stand.

We notice their reluctance, but at the suggestion of a call for backup, we groan inwardly. We make sure that our patient is comfortable and explain that we need to retrieve some equipment before we can help them up from the floor, then head outside to chat with our crew mate. Once in the driveway, out of the patient's earshot, we try to convince our partner that we can manage this lift easily.

They remind us of the patient's history regarding the previous need for lifting equipment. Along with the fact that if either crew member is injured, there will be incident reports to file, recovery time off work, potentially surgical management and ultimately loss of wages should this go wrong. Not to mention the patient's risk of falling if either party become injured mid-way through the lift.

We can't believe it, and we're initially enraged. This partner has been blatantly discouraging safety considerations all day, but they choose now when we just want to get home, to think about such issues?

We cringe, however, when it strikes us that we're no better than they are. Although we hold certain aspects of safety in high regard due to previous incidences we've experienced, or stories that we've heard, we are also happy to push the matter to the back of our mind when it's convenient.

Our partner calmly explains that they are also exceptionally strong and healthy, they have never had a problem with any lift, and they understand our frustration. They also include that it took them a great deal of hard work to get to this stage of their career and fitness goals, therefore they are not willing to jeopardise that, just to save an hour or so of their day.

We look at them with a newfound respect and realise that they feel the same discomfort that we experienced earlier. Simply because of complacency and poor habits that we have picked up along the way, too.

No matter how resilient we think our bodies and minds may be concerning our careers, we are all only one job away from disaster at any given time. The devastating effects of acute injury, chronic illness, violence and motor vehicle incidents may, unfortunately, be unavoidable in some cases, particularly within the paramedic profession.

However, if there are ways that can help to maintain close, unwavering and unashamed focus on prevention, our physical and mental health stands more chance of getting us to retirement, unscathed and capable of enjoying the fruits of our labour. Surely, we owe it to ourselves, and our colleagues, to make this a priority?

The Ugly

Decisions that we make as individual paramedics, regarding our attention to safety, are up to us.

One of the ugliest behaviours, however, has to be when any decision to take unnecessary risk, or blatantly laugh in the face of safety procedures, affects our peers.

Every single one of us will have found ourselves, at some time or other, in the sickening situation of feeling horrified about the danger our crew mates have subjected us to. It's not a pleasant place to be.

THINKING FOR THE TEAM -V- SUITING OURSELVES

We've reached the last night shift of our rotation, and it feels great. One more to go and then days off. We finished late this morning but managed to sleep through the day and turn up a little tired but pretty well-rested.

Our usual partner has taken the night off, so we're waiting for a new crew mate to arrive and start equipment checks. With a blast of loud music and engine revving, we notice a car pulling up one minute before the shift begins. In rushes our colleague for the night, apologising for being late, but they've been out all day catching up with friends and drove straight here.

Energy drink in hand, rapid speech, continual movement, they jump into the driving seat and are raring to go. We are horrified, but do we say something? We tread carefully and ask if they slept at all.

With what appears to be some level of bravado and pride, they start telling us about how busy the last night shift was, but it would take more than that to slow them down, and they have powered through so that they could still go out and play volleyball today with their team, then hang out at the beach.

There's a brief period of hesitation as they realise that we're looking a little shocked, and we suggest that perhaps we switch roles and drive instead, having had a solid six hours of sleep today. They reassure us that everything is okay, nothing to worry about, they do this all of the time, as they line up energy drinks in the pocket of the driver's door.

This example doesn't even need to lead to a story. The story lies at that moment when we realise our partner has no consideration for our safety. Whether it's through naivety, ignorance or arrogance, their social life takes priority over the human body's inbuilt need for rest and recuperation. This colleague is proud of the fact that they've been awake and extremely active for at least twenty six hours and are now about to start a ten to sixteen hour shift.

How can we possibly feel safe in the rear of the ambulance, treating a patient, while they're driving? We can't see whether they can concentrate, make appropriate decisions, or even stay awake.

Working as a team is integral to our profession. Making good personal choices that directly affect our teammates has to form an essential component of that team. Although we may feel indestructible and proud of our stamina, drive and endurance, we must remember to put ourselves in our colleagues' shoes.

If we're behaving in a way that our crew mates question, rather than dismissing that concern, it's vital that we imagine a role reversal. Can we trust this partner with our lives, just as we are expecting them to do with us?

CARING FOR COLLEAGUES -V- REVELLING IN RISK

Against our better judgement, we let it go. Nothing is said. We wanted to push the point, but we also didn't want to create unnecessary tension.

We know that this partner loves high acuity jobs. Their reputation is one of chasing trauma and driving at high speed, but we haven't experienced it firsthand until now.

On the way to a priority call for two patients who have fallen from a height, we are downright terrified. Our partner is whooping with delight, flying through stoplights at intersections.

They notice that we're gripping the handle above the door, to steady ourselves against the sharp turns they're making, and they laugh. We've had enough of saying nothing at this stage. All we can think of is that we just want to get home to our families in one piece by the morning. For some reason, however, politeness and consideration for our crew mate's feelings prevail, and we ask them to slow down because we're feeling unsafe.

Our concern amuses this partner even more. They attempt to goad us into enjoying the ride with advice to "let our hair down" and "stop being so uptight," as this is "the best part of the role."

We are horrified to see another ambulance approaching the intersection just as we reach it, also en route to the nearby patients we're attending. While we're initially relieved to notice that they have slowed down enough to crawl through safely, our partner races through in front of them as if it's a game.

Right then, we decide that it's not. We left it too late to address the situation calmly and begin to shout for them to slow down and stop being so selfish. "Wow!" Comes the reply, as they drop the speed and look across at us. "Everyone said you'd be cool to work with, but you're no fun at all."

As is often the case, ugly behaviour breeds more ugly behaviour. Rather than acknowledge a colleague's concerns or ask themselves why other paramedics don't drive the same way, our crew mate immediately blames us. We wanted to have a conversation about it and explain why we were so concerned, creating an opportunity to rectify the situation, but now, instead, the tension is unmistakable.

As much as the majority of paramedics detest being called "ambulance drivers" we must acknowledge that for around half of our careers, most of us drive an ambulance. (This is not to suggest that the label is fair. It's up to us to educate those who use this term. Opportunities often arise for us to explain our paramedic roles, along with the level of training, education and expertise involved.)

Through this extensive amount of time spent out and about driving, therefore, we are highly visible to other road users, and we are solely responsible for the safe transport of any partner, patient or escort travelling in our vehicle.

This is not a blockbuster movie or high-profile television drama. We are not exempt from the road rules. Although we are provided exceptions in certain emergency circumstances, we remain bound by legislation to make safe driving decisions. Any adverse incident will be dragged into the spotlight for analysis and justification.

Along with the excitement and enjoyment to be derived from driving a vehicle with flashing lights and sirens, exceeding speed limits within reason and utilising areas or directions not traditionally permitted, comes enormous responsibility.

If our driving makes other road users panic, we need to reflect on whether we can change our practices. Should our patients, crew mates and escorts comment negatively, on any aspect of comfort or safety relating to our driving, we must ask ourselves how we can improve. When any partner in the passenger seat appears stressed and feels enough sense of danger, caused directly by our driving, to bring it to our attention, we absolutely must respect that.

There is nothing more inexcusable than laughing at or mocking the fear that we have instilled in others, before continuing to repeat the situation. The personal decisions we make regarding driving risks affect more than just us. Being in the privileged position of operating an emergency vehicle is exactly that, a privilege, not a right; therefore, we must treat it as such.

SOOTHING THE SCENE -V- INCITING THE ANGER

Several calls later, after much awkward silence and being subjected to ridicule for our outburst from our partner's friends as they regaled the story in the ambulance bay, we are travelling to a call for a broken arm.

Our partner hasn't spoken for the entire journey, but we are okay with this, we know it has reached the "point of no return" and just want to just get through the rest of the shift.

While tending to the patient's injuries, information comes to light that their de-facto may have assaulted them. There are empty wine glasses on the kitchen table, a broken lamp on the floor, and it's clear that there has been some kind of altercation. Our partner begins to gain more detail about the incident from the patient's quietly spoken, remorseful looking spouse as we continue our clinical assessment.

The call had been perfectly calm and controlled, despite the tense atmosphere in the room. Still, our crew mate suddenly appears angry at the patient's partner and is raising their voice with an accusation of domestic violence. We feel the agitation rising and suggest to our crew mate that they prepare the stretcher as we finish treating the patient, hoping to remove them from the room so that we can de-escalate the situation.

They refuse. Instead, they fuel the burgeoning fire and become fully engaged in an argument with the alleged offender. The house that we're in now feels hugely unsafe, so we quietly ask the patient to walk outside with us towards the ambulance. Our crew mate begins to follow, along with, as expected, the now angry and aggressive spouse, necessitating an immediate request for police assistance.

Our role is not always easy, particularly when we see behaviours that are upsetting or frustrating to us personally. Colleagues who cause upset or aggression through their behaviour, however, can make it even more difficult. Whether it's inciting argumentative responses from intoxicated patients and bystanders, agitating mental health patients, refusing to back down in a disagreement or something else we may have experienced, this type of situation is fraught with danger.

It is never acceptable to have to tolerate abuse, aggressive or violent behaviour on scene, but there are plenty of occasions when we can rise above poor behaviour directed towards us. Bearing in mind that patients, family members and bystanders are in an emotionally charged situation, having witnessed or been involved in something stressful, often gives us the chance to look at the situation in a different light. Perhaps there are opportunities to calmly and kindly defuse many instances rather than jump in and escalate it further?

Furthermore, we became paramedics to fulfil a vital role and provide care. We don't need to step into the role of police, judge or jury. The more we cross this line, and demonstrate attempts at policing, or judging a situation, the more confusion we create between our roles.

If patients begin to expect us to police their habits, or judge their behaviours, they may react defensively, or with hostility, to our presence.

Many of us take pride in our ability to turn the situation around and avoid escalation, where possible. The ugly behaviour that we're looking at here is the partner who seems to enjoy the confrontation. A partner who goads the domestic violence perpetrator into losing control, knowing that police are there to manage the scene for them. The colleague who takes pleasure in "winding up" our patient, before jumping into the safety of the driving seat, leaving us to deal with the backlash. A partner who chases down the aggressive offender and expects us to assist in wrestling them to the ground.

We need to remember that our manner of dealing with patients is an individual choice. If that choice begins to affect our colleagues negatively, we are now responsible for that reaction, and any disregard for their potential safety must be addressed, no matter how awkward the conversation may feel.

Why It Matters

Arriving home from work, physically and mentally unharmed, is the ultimate goal for every single paramedic on every single shift. A great deal of personal pride is invested in this profession by all of us, particularly with clinical expertise, attention to detail, patient rapport and scene management. Reputation, therefore, plays a huge part in differentiating between the good, the bad and the ugly paramedic.

Without tangible industry benchmarks, monetary objectives or measurable goals, word of mouth reputation becomes the critical indicator of our performance in this line of work. Understandably, it means a great deal to the individual, therefore. We want to enjoy being held in high regard for what we do.

We hear stories about colleagues who performed outstanding accomplishments on difficult calls and their reputation as a good paramedic expands. There may be stories of extremely poor, or what we may consider unnecessary actions, or inactions, which create a reputation more akin to bad paramedic behaviour. How we build, discuss and talk up each other's status, particularly in terms of safety, is both interesting and challenging at the same time.

If we talk about a "crazy driver" colleague with humour and war stories in groups of peers, that reputation becomes accepted as humorous and famously revered.

Does it feel quite as humorous during the shifts that we are travelling in the back, feeling unsafe when there are no friends around to laugh about it with? Why would this colleague choose to change their ways when one brave partner speaks up if all other partners laugh it off?

When we refuse to use the safety harness on the stretcher, and mock other paramedics who always appear to have their patient meticulously secured, we're sending out a clear message that this is acceptable. Why then, would an intern that we're precepting, want to go against this attitude that we have demonstrated throughout the time spent working with them? Surely it makes sense to them that to fit in and gain our respect, they avoid using the safety harness rather than risk our scorn?

Why is it acceptable to use non-complimentary terms such as "overboard," "uptight," "demanding," "stressy," "finicky" and so on when describing a colleague who sticks to the rules and adheres to what we have all been taught? Conversely, why is it not considered equally as acceptable to use terms such as "lazy," "slack," "careless," "irresponsible" or "neglectful" for those who appear to take pride in bending and breaking the rules?

Instead, those types of words are somehow viewed as offensive. We may tend to dress the facts up in terms that sound more palatable, and give others a reason to aspire to, such as "cruisy," "casual," "chilled," "easy-going" and "laid back" for example. It is possible to be the type of paramedic that is relaxed and easy-going to work with, while still maintaining safe practices. Countless paramedics make this look effortless. Unfortunately, there are also countless paramedics, some of them new to the role, who miss the finer details and skip straight to the "chilled" section.

Why would we share memes and promote clothing depicting how paramedics throw caution to the wind as far as safety is concerned, but then expect new colleagues to take what they've been taught seriously?

If we want to be viewed as the "risk-takers" of the medical world, are we sending the message that we take pride in putting our patients, ourselves and our colleagues at risk?

Where did we learn to avoid speaking openly to colleagues when their work choices jeopardise our safety, in favour of valuing their feelings or their opinion of us more highly?

It is possible that in our attempts to avoid hurting a colleague's pride, by saying nothing, we may be complicit in their growing unawareness and blatant disregard.

Put Yourself In The Picture

Think back to the very first time you went out on a shift in an ambulance, and that feeling of overwhelm when you realised just how much there was to pay attention to around you.

Were you acutely aware of safe driving techniques, scene safety, sharp safety, equipment carrying safety, stretcher safety, medication safety, documentation safety and the rest? Where do you sit now in terms of safety considerations, and have you relaxed your initial approach?

How relaxed do you genuinely want your colleagues to be regarding safety when they're working with and around you?

If one of your loved ones was about to step into your work boots and cover your shift, would you want them, or their crew mate, to do anything differently so that they can turn up physically and mentally unharmed the next morning?

As with everything we do in paramedicine, if it's not good enough for our closest family members, then it's not good enough for our patients and, in this instance, it's not good enough for us.

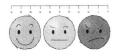

CHAPTER THREE

BEWARE THE BLUFF
BUT WEAR IT WELL

As a general rule, paramedics absolutely must be able to demonstrate on the job confidence to patients, relatives, bystanders, other health professionals, colleagues and often, ourselves, no matter what is happening around us. If we don't, it becomes impossible for us to manage scenes, crowds, situations and clinical treatment, not to mention our natural human reactions.

In the midst of difficult circumstances, to maintain exceptional patient care, through rapid decision making, under pressure, and with little room to falter, confidence is key.

Who hasn't bluffed confidence or quashed intense fear just to get through certain jobs? It's vital that we learn to do this, early and often. We may be looking at a challenging task or confronting sight and thinking "What? This can't be happening!" People rely on us daily to skip past any fears or concerns, so that we can bring out one of the most useful tools in paramedicine...our calm, confident, reassuring demeanour. Our bluff!

For ease of imagination, we can view the bluff as a cloak. When we step into a difficult situation and need to convey calm, reassuring control, we put it on. Wearing the cloak can help us to appear to know what we're doing, even if the reality is that we're floundering around inside. Once the situation becomes safe and ordered, or we've stepped away, off it comes and we hang it up until next time.

In an ambulance environment, however, full of paramedics, it's easy to see just how that bluff can escalate out of control. When surrounded by similar characters, in similar situations, it often leads to a contest of who's the most confident, who knows the most, and who's most in control.

One of the vital skills we are never taught, unfortunately, is how to take that bluff cloak off and put it safely away, until the next time we genuinely need to wear it.

The Good

Whether we've been paramedics for one week or three decades, being receptive to new information and ideas is both vital and humbling all at once. Remember being new and knowing that the paramedic we were working with was doing something "the old way?" Many of us were afraid to tell them about the most recent, easier and safer methods we'd just learnt.

The good paramedic still gets pleasure out of gaining new information because they don't feel any need to wear their bluff, simply to maintain confidence in their skills and knowledge.

Learning new things as we progress, and knowing that we remain adaptable despite our length of service can feel great. It's a true testimony to how good we can be within our roles, and how effortlessly we can remain dynamic and adaptable despite years of experience.

OWNING THE UNKNOWN -V- PRETENDING WE'RE PERFECT

It's the first call of the day, and we're in the attending seat. Our partner has just begun their probationary period, and they're keen to use some of the skills they've learned. Our patient reports momentarily losing consciousness ten minutes ago, and their concerned family members have called an ambulance in case it happens again. We ask our partner to run a twelve lead ECG while we assess the patient's vital signs and immediately notice on the screen that the rhythm looks messy and confusing.

As our partner tears off the printout, they appear perplexed, and the patient asks them how it looks. Being a newer, more junior member of staff, they luxuriously defer to us, telling the patient that we're the ECG expert, so we'll be able to give them a better idea. One glance at the rhythm strip tells us that its interpretation is way out of our skillset. There are some discernible patterns, but it's constantly changing so we can't make head nor tail of the predominant rhythm, but everyone in the room is awaiting our words of wisdom on the subject.

The good paramedic doesn't need to bluff an answer in the hope that we look smart. (Conversely, they also don't play dumb, along the lines of "I'm just a paramedic, so I don't know." As they don't want the patient to feel any sense of sub-standard care.)

We instead say something along the lines of "I don't know what's happening with this rhythm because I haven't seen this pattern before. What I do know is that you've already been unwell this morning, so let's get you off to the hospital and try to get to the bottom of it there."

Humble. Honest. Trustworthy. Professional. Reassuring.

A decisive plan of action is in place.

The patient immediately feels safe in our care and respects that we know exactly what needs to happen. Whether we know the cause or not is likely of little consequence to them at that moment. Their family is relieved to see how seriously the patient's needs are being taken.

Our partner has even more respect for us than before, and they tell us afterwards that it's the first time they have seen such a refreshing approach. No bluff required! They're excited to have found an opportunity to learn something new alongside us, despite our longevity as a paramedic, and this, in turn, increases their self-confidence in not having to put on any bluff.

ASKING THE QUESTION -V- FEARING FOOLISHNESS

Once we arrive at the emergency department, the junior doctor receiving our patient states that they're also confused by the ECG and can't give us a definitive diagnosis. To find out for our own knowledge, as well as our partner's, we wait for the cardiologist to arrive. We ask if it's possible to tag along so that we can listen to their history taking questions and initial diagnostic thoughts, to which they happily oblige.

Our crew mate whispers their concern that the consultant may perceive this as the paramedics not knowing what's going on, and it feels embarrassing.

This provides the perfect chance to explain that it's merely the truth, and we don't know the answer. We can't possibly have a solution for every situation, and neither can any doctor caring for the patient on arrival. It's okay to admit this, it builds trust, and it creates fantastic learning opportunities.

If we bluff our way through any confusion or gaps in knowledge, we run the risk of causing harm and looking completely ridiculous, not to mention dishonest, when it becomes apparent that we were pretending.

Once the cardiologist has finished their assessment, a brief chat highlights a few things. One, they also cannot identify the underlying cause for the patient's unusual arrhythmia; therefore, they intend to continue with tests and various treatments to see if there is any change. Two, their respect for paramedics and our crew dynamic is not only intact, but they compliment us both on the treatment and transport decisions that we've made prior to patient handover. The doctor comments on the great job we do with such limited diagnostic tools in the prehospital setting. Three, our partner learned more from our admission to not knowing, than they would have done had we fobbed them off with a bluffed, fabricated and incorrect answer, just for the sake of our pride.

CREDITING COLLEAGUES -V- CLAIMING THE KUDOS

Later that afternoon, we turn up at a small house at the top of several flights of narrow, rickety stairs and silently hope that the patient can walk to the ambulance. This looks like a logistical, safety nightmare if full stretcher extrication is necessary.

Murphy's Law comes into effect, and the patient needs to be carried to the ambulance, urgently. Our partner calls for backup and organises the necessary equipment while we begin treatment. When the second crew arrives, we give them a quick handover on the patient's condition, and all four paramedics agree on the extrication and treatment plan.

As the safety belts are about to be secured on the extrication board, we quickly reach over and re-position them. They fasten in a different way than usual, decreasing the chance of our patient slipping during a prolonged, steep angled carry down several stairs.

A colleague comments on this ingenuity and the others agree that it's a fantastic idea, highly impressed. Our bluff can make it tempting to accept their praise, and bask in the glory, but our good paramedic drive urges us to share what we've learned. We tell them whom the idea initially came from, and they're no less impressed despite knowing that it wasn't our invention.

Everyone loves to learn new things and, in removing the notion that any paramedic knows everything, we have no hesitation in humbly acknowledging what others have taught us. We don't need to claim ideas as our own or pretend that we already knew information that has only just come to light.

In each of these examples, as with similar situations throughout every shift, if we clear away any romanticism, that one person can be a genius worthy of a pedestal, we create a comfortable arena for knowledge sharing. We remove that interminable pressure to singlehandedly know the answers, and any need to wear our bluff so often, that we begin to forget how to shake it off at all.

The Bad

Over time, as we get more used to our roles, we also become used to knowing more answers, more often. We get comfortable in finding ways to come up with rapid responses, reassure others and build confidence in our presence.

Once we fall into this pattern, the things that we used to have to bluff heavily, become easier to deal with. Situations, or the calls themselves, may not necessarily change, but our reactions to them do.

We find ourselves in limbo between donning the bluff and having it close by. We may not need to wear it so often in terms of our knowledge, now that we know more, but we may inevitably find ourselves wearing it more often.

We become such experts in bluffing, that we can begin to enjoy the way it feels. Less exposed. Less vulnerable. More in control. A favourite item of clothing.

HOSPITABLE HUMOUR -V- MEAN MOCKERY

During the busiest day of the week, we find ourselves rostered to work with a paramedic, who prides themselves on being easy-going, often joking that if they were any more laid back, they'd be horizontal.

We like to think of ourselves as laidback too, but we don't see this as an excuse for cutting corners or taking shortcuts, and we know that working with this person often feels like a battle of wills. We both operate differently. While we are happy to admit when we don't know something and ask questions, they like to appear to know everything, even when we suspect that they don't.

We decide to attend, in the hope that we can maintain best patient care and safety, and our partner tells us that they're happy to drive so that they can kick back and "cruise along" for the day.

On every job, we find our frustration increasing. Each time we update our partner from the back of the ambulance regarding a patient's vitals, we are told that we don't have to keep checking in with our partner, that it's their driving day and we need to have confidence in what we're doing.

When we attempt to countercheck medications before drawing up, we are brushed off with a glance, and the medication remains unconfirmed by our partner. In the guise of establishing rapport and having a jovial conversation with patients and bystanders, it feels like this partner undermines us at every opportunity possible, and it's utterly exhausting.

While attending to an elderly lady with an extensive history of multiple medical conditions, we ask our partner if they can find her medications from the kitchen cabinet. As they call out the brand names, we ask what type of drug one of them is as we don't recognise it, and our partner laughs from the other room, calling out "You're kidding!"

The patient looks a little uncomfortable at the unexpected interaction, but is soon charmed into joining the subtle teasing by our partner when they return to the bedroom and laugh with her about "These paramedics that just don't know their medications."

We're not going to succumb to the pressure and let our ego get in the way, so we look it up and reassure the patient that we understand the medication now that we know its generic name. Explaining that it's unfortunate that brand names often give us no clue, and it's impossible to keep up with the increasing number available on the market.

We know what's happening here, it's all part of the bluff, using humour to distract, reassure and relax our patient. (It's also potentially a way of avoiding having to admit when we don't know the answers ourselves.) It works beautifully on many occasions, and we often come to rely on it as a large part of our treatment.

Some of us, however, rely on it so heavily, that we forget to pay attention to the invisible line. That grey area between the gentle jokes amongst colleagues that demonstrate our collaborative bond to patients, and outright rudeness, condescension and ridicule.

If we're unsure about the tone of our humour, or our partner's, the united front provides our biggest clue. Does the mood portray the crew's unity in caring for the patient together? Or does the bond appear between one paramedic and the patient, as a separate entity from their partner?

En route to hospital, the jibes continue as our partner calls out jokes, and sarcastic comments, from the driving seat to the patient, who laughs along with them and relaxes into the jovial atmosphere. From where we sit, however, our pride begins to hurt. We decide that we'll do everything possible to avoid giving our partner any reason to ridicule us from now on. If we can't beat them, we'll join them.

ENSURING THE EVIDENCE -V- BUILDING THE BLUFF

Around ten hours into the busy shift, we reach our second patient with chest pain for the day. He's an athletic-looking, mid-thirties male, at a local gym, who looks relatively well when we arrive to find him seated on the edge of a weights bench. He tells us that he was working out, felt suddenly out of breath and had some heavy central chest pain, diaphoresis and nausea, lasting several minutes before self-resolving.

The patient's vitals are unremarkable, he is currently completely asymptomatic, and his twelve lead ECG reveals some left ventricular hypertrophy. We state confidently to the patient that this is probably perfectly normal in such an athletic man. He is walking around, gathering his belongings calmly and agrees, saying that he has HCM, so that makes perfect sense to him.

At this stage, we're reluctant to remove our bluff in front of our partner to ask what that abbreviation means, for fear of further ridicule. A glance shows that our partner doesn't look concerned, so we decide to look it up once we enter the ambulance and begin walking the patient towards the vehicle, up several flights of stairs to the parking area.

Once we're seated for transport and on our way, we open up our laptop to begin entering the patient's details, quickly carrying out a surreptitious search for HCM online. A sudden sinking feeling hits us as we realise that keeping our bluff cloak on, purely for ego and pride, could have cost this patient his health, and possibly his life.

We ask how, and when, he found out about his hypertrophic cardiomyopathy while gaining IV access and preparing defibrillation pads in case the situation changes.

The patient informs us that he had a medical last week for an upcoming fitness challenge, but he's not sure what the implications are as the cardiologist appointment is not until later in the week.

We are now aware of the implications, however. We're fully aware of the high risk of sudden cardiac death in such patients and feel frustrated with ourselves. We let our pride get in the way of us asking for clarification on the abbreviated term, so casually thrown into the conversation by our patient.

DROPPING THE ACT -V- BLUFFING TO THE END

Once we've handed our patient over at the receiving hospital, we realise that our partner hasn't commented on the job at all and we're a little surprised. Surely, they must be wondering why we took the precaution of applying defibrillation pads to the patient or did they simply not notice en route as we'd stopped updating them since their previous protestations?

We're faced with the moral and professional dilemma of whether we address the issue and admit our mistake. Our ego wants to let it go and ignore the whole thing. Our sense of professionalism and best patient care knows that we need to bring it up, as a learning opportunity. After the reminder with this most recent patient to swallow our pride and focus on best patient care, we enter the lion's den.

Rather than forcing our partner to admit that they didn't know the abbreviated term for the patient's life-threatening condition by asking "Hey, did you know what he meant when he said HCM?" We say "I had no idea that HCM was an abbreviation for hypertrophic cardiomyopathy, and can't believe I didn't ask him to explain. Lucky he didn't arrest walking up those stairs!"

We want to be good paramedics, and we never want to give up hope that others want the same. We blindly hope that our partner is about to confess that they didn't know either and we can discuss the job we've just finished, openly and honestly. We relish the refreshing opportunity to own up to the fact, together, about our overwhelming desire to wear our bluff like a second skin. Purely to maintain a confident and knowledgeable image, our bluff had the potential to cause our unnecessary patient harm. It doesn't happen though.

Despite the overwhelming suspicion that had our partner known this, they would have seized the opportunity to point out the need to take precautions in case of sudden cardiac arrest, they simply ask "Oh, really?" and laugh in our face.

It stings.

The good paramedic in us thinks of best patient care for the future, and the need to discuss why they didn't mention the danger involved in walking our patient so far. Or the importance of gaining IV access and applying pads in case of arrest. Or any of the other considerations that now seem obvious had they known what the abbreviation meant.

Our inner bad paramedic had sneaked in earlier and now stands taller and more robust at this end of the day. We are tired. We are disappointed that we dropped our usual standards and attempted to fit in with the casual, more complacent approach, purely to avoid ridicule. We know that these thoughts will keep us awake tonight, but we also know that we've learnt a valuable lesson, which certainly won't be repeated.

It's essential for all of us to realise that anyone can adopt bad habits or behaviours at any time. This does not have to make us a bad paramedic through and through.

Most often, we find ourselves doing it just because it's easier. Easier to avoid ridicule. Easier to avoid damaging our pride. Easier to avoid explaining ourselves. Easier to avoid conflict. Easier to avoid upsetting someone. Easier to avoid paperwork. Easier to go with the flow.

The list is probably endless, but whenever we feel that we're taking the path of least resistance more often than not, it's worth looking at it more closely. Assessing whether that path is leading to poor decisions, poor patient care, poor safety, poor professional reputation and ultimately poor self-esteem, poor sleep quality and potentially, poor mental health.

The Ugly

If we have watched paramedic shows originating from around the 1970s and later, we've probably had no idea that we were in many ways attracted to the bluff.

The unspoken confidence boost that appeared to remove any stress from the weird, wonderful and often woeful situations paramedics find themselves in.

For those of us who were taught that "paramedics never run" during our initial training, we understood instantly. In the public eye, running may result in us appearing rushed, out of breath and quite possibly out of control.

Our bluff cloak would fall off.

If this happened, we would have no value in calming a stressful scene.

What happens when we begin to wear it as a second skin and forget how to take it off?

ENLIGHTENING EDUCATION -V- STAYING STAGNANT

It's a sunny Sunday morning, and our shift began with a leisurely coffee rather than an early job. What a great start! Our attending partner for the roster is an experienced paramedic whom we know relatively well, so we've slipped into a comfortable routine for the day after attending to a couple of patients already.

When we're ramped at a large hospital, several crews are waiting in the corridor, so the conversation soon turns to continued professional development. We're quite comfortable with this, and it's a suitable topic to have around patients who are resting and being attended to by the crews they arrived with. When the subject of researching complicated cases comes up, it's interesting to hear how other paramedics manage their education.

Some are relaying their need to rely on individual learning styles by listening to reputable podcasts, reading articles, signing up for conferences, watching evidence-based videos online and more. It's surprising, therefore, to hear our partner state, with great conviction, that they have been in the role for long enough that they don't need to do the "extra work" any longer.

A little stunned silence follows.

Another paramedic asks what they mean, to which our partner replies that they "know their stuff." They've been a paramedic for several years and state "Once you've seen one chest pain, you've seen them all!"

A discussion ensues in which several paramedics, some of whom have been employed for considerably longer than our partner, unashamedly state that the longer they are in the role, the more they realise just how much there is to learn and how rapidly evidence-based practice is changing. Our partner disagrees, however. They are adamant that they know enough. While they agree that they'll do enough to tick the boxes, solely for the obligatory annual continual professional development, they feel confident that their experience outweighs everything else.

We are astounded at this thought process. Looking around, we see that there are paramedics involved in the conversation with an entire lifetime of experience. Still, they are happily aware that they need and want to continue to learn on an ongoing basis for best patient care. They casually mention several areas that they want to research in more detail, without embarrassment, clearly proud to admit that they can't know everything.

A couple of new interns appear to be impressed by our partner's point of view, however and are nodding their heads in appreciation. Clearly swayed by the confident delivery and self-belief our partner has in their skills and knowledge. All of a sudden, a nurse calls out our patient's name, and we are allocated a bed, so we wheel our stretcher through to the department for handover.

Nothing. Goes. Wrong.

At least, not in this example, or this chapter, but we know it will!

Although we have seen some complacency and possibly arrogance in this partner before, we now realise that they wear their bluff so tightly that they feel invincible in their role.

No room for improvement through looking at other practices, as they rely on their bluff to convince themselves that they don't need to improve.

No room for learning by self-reflection. This paramedic believes their bluff to such a degree that the idea of self-reflection is out of the question.

No room for taking other opinions and evidence on board, as such a suffocating bluff prevents them from hearing anything that may bring their thoughts, ideas or beliefs into question.

The only thing that their bluff is protecting, however, is their ego, and unfortunately, once we've seen this in a colleague, it's hard ever to view them in the same light.

TREATING THE CALL -V- JUSTIFYING JUDGEMENT

Once we're clear from the long wait in the hospital, we are en route to a call for a teenager in cardiac arrest at a local skate park. Our partner begins to recount stories about the worst "fake" cardiac arrest they have ever witnessed. At the roadside, we are waved down by onlookers, who direct us across the grass, towards a teenaged patient lying in the lateral position, surrounded by friends. Our partner strolls across to the patient and kneels to check their pulse, attempting to gain a response by calling out as well as shaking the patient's shoulder, without success.

They appear to be breathing, and our partner tells us that they have a strong, regular carotid pulse, but the patient still isn't responding. Bystanders tell us that the patient sat down on the grass and stated that they felt unwell, before slumping sideways, at which point an ambulance was called.

As instructed by the call taker, CPR was commenced and then stopped after around two minutes, when the patient began moaning and pushed the first aid providers away. Upon hearing this, our partner delivers a sharp, aggressive sternal rub to the patient, which rouses them with a yelp and their eyes open.

We begin to open the treatment bag and cardiac monitor while this is going on, in preparation for assessment and pre-emptive management, but our partner whispers to us that the patient is "faking it" and shakes their head at the equipment we're opening up. They declare to the group that the patient is young, fit and healthy, more than likely just fainted, and needs to get up and walk over to the ambulance.

We find ourselves suddenly in that familiar and awkward "no man's land" between protecting the patient's best interests and protecting our partner's reputation. Do we speak up and voice our concerns that we can't dismiss what the bystanders are saying, in case the patient genuinely did arrest and is now in a fragile, post-cardiac arrest state? Do we keep quiet to save embarrassing our partner and just assume that their dismissive attitude is correct?

We know, in our heart of hearts, that we just can't let this go. We have enough education and experience to understand that ignoring the information available is putting our patient at risk. Treating this as a post-cardiac arrest call, and taking the necessary precautions, will be a whole lot easier than ignoring the history and having them crash on us.

Who cares if they're faking it? We're not willing to risk our patient's health, or our career just to be proven correct.

We quietly lean down to our partner and ask if we can have a quick word, gesturing towards the ambulance. Instantly, their body language changes as they look us in the eye, and we feel sick to the pit of our stomach, at the thought of the potential confrontation we're about to face. As soon as we're out of general earshot, our partner demands to know "What's the matter?"

We aim to soothe the situation by meeting halfway and start with comments around how we agree that it's all probably fake. We suggest that maybe it would be better, in full view of so many bystanders, if we took the precautions we'd usually take in any other post-cardiac arrest call, just in case. They laugh mockingly and tell us "not to stress" and "stop overtreating" with reassurances that they've seen this dozens of times and the patient is definitely faking it.

We can't risk conceding this point. We just know, that gut feeling is there that it's simply the wrong thing to do. So, we resort to justifying that they're probably right, but it would make us feel better if we can exercise all precautions, purely to avoid any hassle if something goes wrong.

Surprisingly, they give in. With a laugh and a cynical shake of the head, they agree, and the patient is transported with great care and attention. During the drive there, we are frustrated and annoyed with ourselves for failing to call out such complacent and careless behaviour. Instead, we sold the idea as if we were nervous, or stressed and that it was purely to appease us, rather than risk questioning their judgement.

Ugly behaviour in all walks of life often seems to carry more volume and weight than the good it opposes. Possibly due to its shock value, the fact that it feels confrontational, its ability to hurt feelings, the way it can shake confidence and so on.

In paramedicine, this type of behaviour often rears its ugly head if there is any threat to the bluff that can be worn so casually over time. Any suggestion of taking a different approach may elicit a harsh response. The questioning of an individual's ideas, opinions or approach can ignite a volatile reaction. Rather than work as a cohesive time, shut down becomes the best default mechanism in defending self-pride and strengthening the illusion of being in control.

Every single one of us has likely experienced a similar situation countless times. While our paramedic partner probably started their career with the best of intentions, their overwhelming desire to appear cool, calm and collected has now completely enveloped their character. This may render them unwilling and often unable to see the value in working as a team, with shared ideas, towards best patient care. Preferring instead to push their opinions and views upon others and make fun of those wishing to do the right thing.

We are aware that with some colleagues, it's possible to discuss this, and there is plenty of value in doing so. We are also mindful, however, that sometimes, our bluff has been worn so tightly, for so long, that it has become our second skin and can no longer be removed. The only choice we're left with, in these situations, therefore, is to stand up and be heard in favour of best patient care. In doing so, we are risking the wrath of a colleague who is intent on being right, rather than doing the right thing.

One question that arises on such occasions, however, that we must ask ourselves internally, is that of our own behaviour. Does our refusal to advocate for best patient care, just to avoid confrontation or upsetting our partner, make our practice equally ugly, only in a more insidious way?

EMBRACING ERRORS -V- BELIEVING OUR BLUFF

After shaking off the nagging frustration in ourselves and ending the shift without incident, we head home for the night and manage to leave all thoughts of work behind us.

The next morning, however, we arrive at work to find an ambulance manager waiting for us with a clipboard full of notes. Never a good sign!

Our partner is sitting at the table with the manager, looking quite relaxed and comfortable, so we're not too concerned. It turns out that our case resulted in a complaint from a member of the public, unhappy that their concerns were not taken seriously. They were extremely upset at the dismissive behaviour of the attending paramedics after the patient had been in cardiac arrest and was fortunately revived by those rendering first aid on scene.

Upon auditing the patient care record, it transpires that the interventions and on-scene times differed significantly from that expected for a post-cardiac arrest patient. Subsequent follow up with the hospital revealed that the patient was diagnosed with long Q-T syndrome, with pacemaker implantation scheduled to occur, before they could be discharged home.

Our partner looks up and exclaims "That explains everything!" Going on to talk at length about how they knew something had been seriously wrong, but couldn't quite put their finger on it at the time. They comfortably regale the story of how difficult it had been to gain information at the scene, and now begin to bring us into the conversation.

Quite convincingly, our partner describes the call as if we had both been on the same page and of the same opinion, investigating all differential diagnoses thoroughly. We sit, in silent shock, at what we are hearing.

Once the manager has left, we turn to our partner and make a light-hearted comment about how convincing their version of events was. We are even more horrified by their response. "I knew there was more to that patient than meets the eye."

They are serious! Their interpretation has them totally convinced of the events surrounding the case. It wasn't an act of whitewash to avoid disciplinary action as we initially suspected.

Their bluff has rendered them utterly unreceptive to suggestion, oblivious to reason, impervious to judgement and skilled in believing their selective interpretations of events. They cannot remove their bluff, it is no longer a useful garment, but instead an irremovable second skin.

Why It Matters

Learning to create a sense of calm as soon as we arrive on scene is vital in paramedicine. Maintaining our cool and ensuring effective control is an art. One which we must become skilled in rapidly if we are to remain safe and carry out quality emergency medical care in every random situation we face. We also work in a highly competitive profession and are therefore also forced, right from the beginning, to find ways that give us an edge. We have to excel, in a manner recognisable enough to secure a successful career.

If we think about it logically, right from the beginning, there are very few ways to prove how good we are, to get hired, until we start working in an ambulance on road.

We can learn great interview techniques to help clear our path through hundreds or thousands of competitors towards winning a coveted role.

We can practice scenario exercises endlessly until we outperform other applicants by appearing calm, professional and slick in simulated assessments.

We can study hard and excel academically so that we stand out from the crowd on paper and by word of mouth.

Some paramedics manage to do all three, but what happens once we've secured our dream role? The bluff happens!

It is invaluable in protecting patients, stressed bystanders, ourselves and our colleagues through the confidence it helps to convey in our decision-making skills, even when we may be highly stressed and unsure on the inside. Wrapping ourselves in the bluff gives us the courage to try new skills and test out our training when required, even if we'd be quaking in our boots without its protection. It is vital in providing us with the necessary steady demeanour to direct multiple agencies and personnel on scene during times of crisis.

Most importantly, on those occasions where we are under direct threat, the addition of this invisible cloak of armour may be enough to help us raise ourselves just a little taller. To push out our chests just a little further and use just a little more volume in standing our ground.

If we had known the damage that this continual need to bluff could do to our personality and character traits before becoming paramedics, however, we may have insured ourselves against its overpowering ability to gain the upper hand earlier. Unlike a physical uniform, it's not so easy to recognise whether we've removed the bluff when it's no longer required.

The more often we have to wear it, the better it fits, and the more comfortable it becomes. We may want to wear it more often, only because it feels so good. Perhaps we wear it constantly at work because it's what makes us most comfortable. Potentially we begin wearing it in social situations, for that additional confidence boost. Maybe we even wear it in all aspects of our personal lives, because taking it off makes us feel vulnerable.

Once it remains stuck, however, the only thing it protects is our ego, and it begins to create the opposite effect, putting those we initially sought to protect, at risk.

In the same manner, the protection it once provided us with can render us prisoners. If we use it too often, it may begin to suffocate potential growth throughout our careers and personal lives.

Any refusal to remain open to listening to others, recognising gaps in knowledge, considering suggestions regarding better ideas or making room for improvement, leaves us stuck right where we are. From here, we risk being left behind or making grave errors in judgement.

Removing the bluff and listening with fresh ears for things that make us question, and challenge, and learn, keeps us in touch with change and more vigilant in maintaining excellent patient care.

As soon as we develop tunnel vision by refusing to look at the bigger picture because our bluff blinds us, we run the risk of tripping up and falling into unnecessary trouble. Taking off that bluff cloak, and opening our eyes fully, gives us the peripheral vision necessary to notice not only the potential perils and pitfalls but the treasures and rewards to be gained from great working relationships, that we'd otherwise miss.

Aside from our professional environment, wearing that bluff home will undoubtedly expose us to the same risks, but with adverse effects on ourselves, our families, friends, teammates and loved ones. If we can no longer listen openly, recognise the ideas of others, embrace new challenges, see where we may be going wrong, reveal our authentic voice, thoughts or vulnerabilities, we become a shell of the person we once were. Perhaps our families are the best judges of how well we drop the bluff when we step over the threshold of our homes.

Put Yourself In The Picture

When you first began toying with the idea of working in an ambulance, did you want to be the type of paramedic that was renowned for being motivated, always learning new things, open to new ideas and enthusiastic? Or did you want to be known as dismissive, arrogant, unwavering and obstructive in your role?

Remember the paramedics you met when you were new, to whom your colleagues referred when they talked about innovative and inspirational practitioners? Do you recall watching people approach them to ask questions, obtain advice or seek opinion, and feel impressed not only by their knowledge but by their comfort in stating when they didn't know or weren't sure of, the answer?

Think about how comfortable you found it to be open about any gaps in your knowledge, hopes for the future, and your willingness to learn when you first became a paramedic. Is it still as easy for you now, or do you prefer to hide any chinks in your confident armour instead?

Check for that bluff when you're not in a high-pressure situation. If you find you're wearing it so often that you've lost yourself along the way, give yourself a break and practice taking it off in safe situations. Practice saying, "I don't know" and enjoy the chance to learn new things from your family, friends and colleagues.

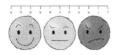

CHAPTER FOUR

PRECEPTING PARAMEDICS FOR OUR OWN OLD AGE

Mentoring, or precepting, new paramedic students and interns is a huge responsibility and privilege and should be treated as such. Often, it's possible to tell who a new paramedic's first preceptor was, purely by their behaviour on calls, be it good, bad or ugly.

At other times, it may be surprising to find out which paramedic initially precepted a new staff member, because the intern has gone out of their way to avoid mirroring behaviours that they've recognised as undesirable, or unacceptable, in their practice.

There are exceptions to the rule, but most interns have very little exposure to an ambulance environment before they step into our care. They may have attended some ridealongs, they may have volunteered in a first responder capacity, and they may have watched plenty of television shows depicting what we do.

The first roster or rotation in their hands-on role, however, is critical in shaping the clinical practice and professional behaviour of colleagues who may one day turn up at our own homes in times of crisis. The standard of care that we'd like our families to receive, therefore, potentially lies in our hands.

The Good

When it comes to precepting, we walk a very thin line. The need to empower an intern is vital in having them learn through real experience.

At the same time, however, we must prevent them running ahead before they can walk alongside us, to avoid patient harm and the development of poor clinical or behavioural habits.

There are ways, however, that the good paramedic can remain well balanced on that precariously thin line, all while facilitating an expanse of learning for the preceptee in our charge.

SETTING UP FOR SUCCESS -V- CONSTANT CONFUSION

As soon as we arrive at work early one morning for our first shift, we meet our newly allocated intern partner. After quick introductions around the ambulance station, we manage to spend almost an hour going through the vehicle and equipment checks, highlighting where everything is, and how to find it quickly. Surprisingly, no job has yet been allocated to our crew, so we continue with our plan to familiarise the intern with as many essential aspects as possible before we get caught up in the chaos that sounds prevalent over the airwaves.

We use this opportunity to take them for coffee and, during our chat, bring up the subject of expectations, asking what they want, and need, to get out of this roster together. They have a list and give us a rundown of what they've been told are strong points, as well as the weaker points they'd like to improve upon. It's a great start. We let them know what our expectations are, in clear and direct language, and explain how we intend to communicate openly, no matter what the feedback. They visibly relax into their seat just a little, feeling better prepared for the day ahead.

Without this time to familiarise a preceptee on their very first shift, they may likely feel as if they're floundering around, in a constant state of confusion, until they've worked out the logistics for themselves. (Although it's not always possible to facilitate this time to acclimatise, it's important to remember that, without it, they may have little idea about the equipment, storage locations, our precepting style or expectations.)

During this phase of high alert, rather than concentrating on tasks that come up, an intern's focus may be stuck on second-guessing what we could be thinking, or about to say, as they have no idea what their preceptor expects from them. They may find it impossible to locate essential items in the ambulance on pressurised calls, simply because the haze of confusion makes them rush, and blindly panic. They may avoid asking questions when it's vital that they do seek clarification, purely out of fearing the unknown, that is the paramedic preceptor they feel the need to impress.

Despite such a pleasant start to the shift, we are inevitably tasked to a job eventually, so it's perfect timing when we receive a call to back up a crew on a drug overdose.

En route to the scene, we run through our primary and secondary surveys, as well as medication dosages and the importance of effective ventilation. Our partner seems pretty switched on and, despite sounding a little nervous, they appear to have a good grasp of what needs to happen. With a sudden shift in focus, they begin to ask questions about how we know what to look for when approaching stop signs and intersections while driving on lights and sirens, but we tell them that we'll be happy to run through all of that later. For now, we plan to only talk about the call we're about to work on, without distraction, so that they can focus on best patient care and safety.

Once the job is over, the primary crew begin transporting their now conscious patient to the emergency department. After cleaning up the scene and returning to our ambulance, we explain that we'll take care of the patient care report, and we'd like them to make a list of everything they did or saw on the job that they thought was great, or anything that they feel could have been done differently and why.

Through this list, we have the chance to gain a little insight into the level of care our preceptee may be capable of giving. We're pleasantly surprised to find that they had observed the end tidal capnography reading as soon as we arrived, and counted the rate at which the patient was being ventilated.

This provides us with the chance to praise them for such significant attention to detail rather than being distracted by the confronting scene itself.

They ask why the initial attending crew didn't travel on a priority one upon leaving the scene despite the patient's poor condition. A golden opportunity to talk about how such decisions are made upon patient presentation rather than the scripted format that needs to be used in initial training.

They don't mention the discarded sharps around the house, so we ask what their thoughts are, and they are surprised to find that they didn't notice, leading to a useful discussion around safety awareness on scene.

After making it clear that we are in no way judging the attending crew's care, and are only using it as a realistic scene to overview, it proves to be a valuable exercise for both of us. Our intern agrees that while they were initially disappointed at not being the attending crew, having slightly less involvement, as the backup crew, has provided them with a much broader learning experience. We have managed to gain a feel for their overall insight capabilities, rather than being limited to only hands-on involvement in patient care.

SAFETY NET SUPPORT -V- RULING THE ROOST

Once we're finished with our paperwork and debriefing, dispatch notifies us that there are no outstanding calls and we don't argue with this unusual state of affairs, as we drive towards our base. Just around the corner, however, an ambulance has been called to a convulsing patient. We are allocated the job and arrive almost immediately, without time to discuss a management plan in advance.

We make it clear that our partner is running the call before stepping out of the vehicle and reassure them that they can be confident in knowing that we will step in if necessary. A quiet reminder that their observations and considerations from the last call already prove that their training has prepared them well, empowers them to walk towards the patient's front door with confidence.

As soon as we enter the kitchen of the property, it's clear that the patient is still in the throes of a generalised seizure. They are thrashing around, grunting, foaming at the mouth and have been incontinent. Family members quickly inform us that this is a regular occurrence, and despite the increased frequency lately, nothing else about it is unusual. Our patient was lowered to the floor without trauma immediately when the seizure began, and they have been placed on their side in a safe area until it subsides.

We look across at our partner to make sure that they've taken this information on board and notice that they appear shocked at the scene before them. We remember that no amount of simulated exercises, medical videos or textbooks can prepare us for the sight and sound of up-close experiences, and bring them back to the task with a gentle hand on the shoulder, quietly asking what their plan is.

It seems to do the trick. The human contact and quiet request help them to regain control of their thoughts and they quickly establish, in a friendly and direct manner, from family members, the timing, usual medications and type of management that is generally required when the patient convulses. With this information on board, our intern outlines their plan for benzodiazepines, airway management, monitoring and extrication like a pro. Instilling a great sense of calm and control for the family as they stand by, feeling helpless until the patient regains consciousness.

UPSKILLING WITH CARE -V- ASSUMING INEPTITUDE

After administering medication, full assessment, oxygenation, gaining IV access, drawing blood and assisting the now post-ictal patient in getting cleaned up and into fresh clothing for transport, we find ourselves settling into the ambulance when the patient begins to convulse again on the stretcher. Our partner is quick to suggest moving the patient into a lateral position to protect their airway, and we tell them that it's a fantastic idea, assisting them in unstrapping the harness, moving the patient and re-securing them safely.

This seizure does not last very long, but our patient is still barely conscious, so we mention to our partner that we are keen to get to a hospital quickly, as we are probably dealing with status epilepticus. We suggest that it would be great to secure basic airway adjuncts for now and we can consider more definitive measures en route should they prove necessary.

Our partner measures and attempts to place an oropharyngeal airway, but discovers intermittent trismus, and they cannot insert the device into the patient's mouth. We reach out to hand them a pre-prepared nasopharyngeal airway instead, but they look visibly stressed and ask if we can insert it for them so that we can get moving.

Having had a brief overview of our intern's knowledge, thought processes and abilities already this morning, we decide that they are probably highly capable of inserting the NPA. Still, their confidence is wavering, and they need a little boost. We use this opportunity, to refresh that confidence, place the airway device in their hand decisively and talk them through the skill until, twenty seconds later, it's in situ and we're ready to go.

En route to the hospital, we can feel a sense of achievement and pride emanating from our partner. They call out updated A-E findings at regular intervals, make fantastic suggestions regarding pre-emptive measures that they're preparing for in case of deterioration and then deliver their bedside handover beautifully on arrival, without faltering, before stepping outside to begin the patient report paperwork.

It's such a satisfying transition to watch. We grow to enjoy being a part of those moments of faltering confidence, during which we weigh up whether we think the intern is capable and just needs a boost to overcome the mental hurdles involved in new or challenging skills. Or whether it's in the patient's best interests for us to take over instead.

In this instance, our partner is delighted when we chat about it. They have completed their first airway intervention successfully and say that now it won't feel so daunting in future. Their confidence in their abilities has improved, and they feel safe in the knowledge that we will calmly overview their management, nudging them in the right direction if necessary but ready to step in as soon as the patient's requirements change.

This type of support is exactly where the fine line exists. All the while that we can quietly work alongside our partner without jumping in to take over or interrupting their flow to ask questions just to suit our own systematic approach, they are learning their craft. Sometimes they'll do it well and feel great about it. Other times, they might do a terrible job and, as long as the patient will not suffer any adverse consequence in any way, the best thing we can do is let them stumble. Providing them opportunities for self-reflection and, ultimately, self-improvement.

The Bad

In some ambulance services, it may be compulsory to precept new members of staff. In others, we may have to apply or be nominated for that role. In most, at some point, we will work with volunteers, students and interns, as well as paramedics who are still relatively new in their careers.

In each of these situations, our individual clinical practices and behaviours are observed continuously for shifts lasting between eight and twenty four hours. It's very easy, therefore, to forget about the good intentions we may have had during our precepting periods and fall into bad habits, modelling them as options to those who are looking to us for guidance.

CONSCIENTIOUS CARE -V- DROPPING OUR DILIGENCE

As soon as we wake up in the late afternoon for the night shift ahead, we're hit with that feeling of dread. We can hear our family laughing and chatting outside, music playing, and the delicious smell of a barbeque filtering through the house. We get up and shower, preparing for work, but feel resentful at missing out on the weekend fun, grabbing some food from the counter and heading off in the car to start our shift.

We haven't got much to say for ourselves, and we struggle to cope with the enthusiasm and energy of our intern who seems to love doing everything by the book, even though we've suggested a few shortcuts. Around midnight, we can no longer tolerate the mess they make and the amount of equipment they use because it's our turn to drive, and we are sick of wiping down and re-stocking.

The next call we attend is a middle-aged gentleman with abdominal pain. He's waiting at the front door, with a bag packed, when we pull up in the driveway. We leave the engine running and encourage our partner to have him walk over to the ambulance and sit in the seat.

He looks a little pale and diaphoretic, so our partner asks him to lie on the stretcher, but we interrupt from the door of the ambulance and tell him to stay where he is seated, as he tells us about the pain. He describes it as generalised discomfort across his stomach. It's been there on and off all day. He has type two diabetes, is overweight and has no other history.

We reassure our partner that the patient is fine where he is and brush off their gesture towards applying the cardiac monitor. As soon as the patient has his seatbelt on and our partner is beginning to assess his vitals, we move to the cab, put on some favourite music, drive towards the emergency department and safely deliver our patient into the triage area.

Our mood has lifted a little. We have no equipment to wipe down and pack away, nothing to re-stock, no stretcher to clean and make up with linen, so we chat with some colleagues and enjoy a little time to surf the internet.

While waiting, we see that our patient has been placed on a bed and wheeled into the resuscitation bay. So we follow our partner through to find out what's going on. It turns out that the patient has a silent MI and our partner looks horrified. As we shuffle out, they ask whether we'll be in trouble for not assessing our diabetic patient further.

We don our bluff and confidently reassure them that the patient had no chest pain and, we're not doctors, so we can't be expected to look for everything in every single patient. We can only do the best with what we have, and we have fulfilled our primary duty by transporting our patient to definitive care. We're relieved to find that they're happy with this justification, and the subject is dropped. Our shift goes on to end without incident, and we head home for days off, and the much needed catch up with family.

Often, we don't have to do bad things to behave like a bad paramedic. Cutting down on the level of service we provide, however, when we have the means and the education to assess for well-known possibilities, certainly doesn't feel like we're doing the best within our role.

We may be able to convince ourselves that it does, but on any occasion where we find that justification is required, the clues are there, letting us know that maybe our standards are slipping.

EQUAL STANDARDS -V- PRIORITISING OUR PREFERENCES

Around six months later, we're working with this partner once again, as they near the end of their intern year. We are dispatched to a job at an address we recognise, a recently retired friend. We're not too concerned as the call states that they have abdominal pain, and we tell our partner some funny stories about camping trips we've been on together.

When we arrive, our patient is sitting in a dining chair, looking slightly pale and grimacing. We chat with them, while our attending partner checks their blood pressure and oxygen levels, before suggesting that the patient walks out to the ambulance so that we can take them to hospital for assessment.

We're a little surprised that they don't assess a blood glucose level, grab the cardiac monitor and run an ECG, or at least a three lead, as they're usually so thorough, but we're not too perturbed at this stage and stroll out to the vehicle with our friend. When our partner gestures towards the seat, we look over in surprise and suggest that perhaps the stretcher would be best. They dismiss us, and close the door, ready for transport.

We stand outside for a second, caught between letting it go and voicing our concerns. Our training and experience tell us that there may be more to the abdominal pain. If there's something more serious happening with our friend, we don't want to miss the opportunity to intervene early, if it means helping them towards a positive outcome.

Instinct tells us, however, that re-opening the door and requesting our partner change their management plan may cause some awkwardness for the remainder of the shift. Friendship overrules. We risk the potential conflict, open up the doors and ask if our partner would mind placing the patient on the stretcher and carrying out a twelve lead, just to be on the safe side.

They don't react poorly to the suggestion and, other than a slight raise of the eyebrows, they look happy to oblige. Nothing shows up on the ECG, our patient remains relatively comfortable, and it later turns out that he has chronic constipation, before being discharged home with laxative medication.

After handover, our partner asks why we felt it was essential to carry out full cardiac monitoring and utilise the stretcher. We begin to explain the risks of missing the more serious causes of abdominal pain, and the importance of using diagnostic equipment even in the absence of chest pain. There is a period of silence. We feel that our explanation is logical and clinically sound. Still, the realisation suddenly hits us when they ask why this call differed from the cardiac case we missed several months ago.

We, quite possibly along with other preceptors, have been responsible for teaching our partner to drop their excellent standards. We actively discouraged them from assessing for less obvious signs and symptoms. We actively encouraged them to place patients sitting up, to avoid using the stretcher, as often as possible. We dismissed their attempts at providing the highest standards of care on so many occasions during our last run of calls together.

Now, however, just because our patient is a personal friend, we expected that standard to change. It feels bad. We didn't set out to behave badly in this role, and it hurts our pride to make this realisation.

ADMITTING THE ERROR VS COVERING UP WITH CONTEMPT

The shift continues, nothing is said, but the elephant remains in the room. We sense growing sarcasm from our partner, asking if we'd prefer to transport a trauma patient seated or on the stretcher. Joking with a cardiac patient that we'll only apply the monitor if we like them, and suggesting that the pain scale is only valid if the patient is a friend or relative.

At this point, it has become evident that we need to heed the good paramedic we hear internally and face up to a brave, open and honest conversation. We need to clear the air, as well as, most importantly, highlight the dangers of taking shortcuts, despite our previous poor advice.

The bad paramedic option is more appealing, however, because our pride is at risk and we feel as if we're losing credibility. The moment is lost as we suddenly snap and attempt to reinstate our authority over the intern.

While attending to a patient with a chest infection, they connect the wrong size of nasal prongs to the oxygen cylinder. We know it doesn't make a difference, they're still pointing up into the patient's nostrils, and flow is not affected, they're merely smaller and don't sit so well in situ.

Rather than let it go and avoid discrediting our partner, or making our patient doubt the quality of care they're receiving, we joke about the "newbie" instead. Our ego has encouraged us to embarrass our partner rather than face our discomfort around the double standards we demonstrated earlier in the shift. The damage is done.

The valuable opportunity to admit our error in judgement, and create a positive lesson for both parties, has been lost. Worst of all, however, is that we have allowed poor clinical behaviours, and an unacceptable style of precepting, to become familiar in this paramedic's toolbox for the future.

We can find ourselves behaving badly, even when it's not intentional. Saving face, adopting a few lazy habits, attempting to avoid embarrassment, and being unwilling to admit to poor decisions can quickly make a bad paramedic out of a good one.

Whatever we put out as an example, we must expect to see reflected back at us in new paramedics as they progress, and, ultimately, in the interns that they will precept in the future.

The Ugly

Once we start to succumb to bad paramedic behaviour, the width of the gap between bad and ugly reduces in line with our level of exposure. The more we practice bad habits, the better we get at them. The more shortcuts we get away with, the more likely we are to stick with the easiest option.

For some new paramedics, but not all, spending an entire roster or prolonged period with a bad, or ugly paramedic, can be enough to shape similar habits, no matter how much they were opposed to this type of behaviour in the beginning.

DISCOURAGING DILIGENCE -V- CURATING COMPLACENCY

We've recently taken on the role of preceptor. Having never worked with an intern before, we are slightly nervous. We're a little unsure of our capabilities in attending any big jobs when we're only accompanied by a brand new staff member, with no experience to fall back on. We don't want to mention our concerns to anyone else, they might think less of us and doubt our confidence, so we rely on our bluff instead.

Our intern arrives, and we show them around the station. We dismiss their attempts at checking the ambulance, telling them that we've done a quick "embarrassment check" and explain that this covers the absolute basics. Anything else that's missing isn't critical. They look a little uncomfortable, but they're new.

"They'll get the hang of it soon enough." We tell ourselves, as we head out to the vehicle and see our colleagues checking their equipment in preparation for the shift. After introducing our intern to the group and making jokes about how new their uniform looks, we laugh about how much fuss the other crew make with their ambulance checks.

Our partner appears to relax visibly. We can see them adopting a more comfortable stance, hands in pockets, leaning against the ambulance in a carefree pose, quickly picking up on how casual and easy-going we appear to be in our paramedic role.

Nobody, in our opinion, wants to look fixated on checking equipment, keeping everything clean and re-stocked. That doesn't convey a sense of calm and control, that just looks like a new paramedic, too keen!

During the drive to the first call of the day, our partner attempts to ask us how we like to work, and whether we have any particular preferences. They've been advised to do this in training so that they can work optimally with different paramedics who may have specific ways of doing things. We laugh and tell them "Don't stress. Just go with the flow!" Emphasising how laid back we are. We explain that things are very different in the real world than they are in a training college.

What we haven't realised is that we are using so many clichés that we're beginning to sound like one. We're so desperate to put an air of confidence out there that we mistake the intern's visible shift in stance and attitude as them relaxing. In all likelihood, they're simply making every attempt to fit in.

By ridiculing the professional behaviour of others, in order to look casual, we're teaching our new partner that they'll be laughed at if they try to do the right thing. Through dismissing the safety net of the preparation techniques they were trained to rely upon, we remove every tool that the intern felt armed with upon arriving. Now they're stuck in limbo, between the systematic preparation that multiple tutors, lecturers, textbooks and evidence-based teaching provided, and our nonchalant approach.

RESPECTING THE RULES -V- TRAINING FOR TROUBLE

After arriving and assessing our patient, while preparing to draw up some morphine, our partner holds out the vial, asking us to check the medication. We wave it away, indicating that we don't need to check it. They persist. They ask again if we can check the drug name and expiry date.

We're busy gaining IV access and reassure our partner that we trust them, and to just draw it up, so they do. They hand us a labelled syringe upon which they've written the dilution under the medication name. We administer it.

Nothing goes wrong.

We're dispatched to several calls. Multiple drugs are drawn up. Nothing goes wrong. The next job requires naloxone in a hurry, so we tell our partner to forget about the labels and writing down the solution concentration, it all takes too long, and we have essential interventions to perform.

A crew backs us up on a cardiac arrest call, and every time one of the paramedics prepares adrenaline, they show the vial to their partner and ask them to check it before drawing it into a labelled syringe. The intern glances at us with a slight raise of the eyebrows.

We laugh about it together afterwards, how pedantic that paramedic is, how they always have to do everything by the book and they're no fun to work with. We reason that it takes so long to do all of the checks, draw up the medication, write up labels and seal the syringe with a cap that as soon as one is administered, it's time to start the whole process again in preparation for the next dose.

The next day, it's our partner's turn to attend. They don't even ask us to check medications today, we just draw up what they ask for, and they push it. Things are flowing smoothly. The day is progressing well.

This intern is great, despite how new they are, they seem to know what they're doing, and we're getting things done to an incredibly high standard. During one call, we hand them an unlabelled syringe containing an opioid, as well as one containing saline, but the saline flush still has the plastic ampoule on the end of it, so it's obvious to us which is which.

They administer half of one syringe and then flush with the full contents of the other before realising that they aren't sure which was which. They are a little worried that they may have pushed a full syringe of opioids, followed by a smaller saline flush in error, but we talk about it afterwards at length.

We discuss that these things can't be helped, we're under a lot of pressure on chaotic scenes, and it's completely unavoidable. We also reassure them that with opioids, we can always reverse any error with naloxone, so they feel a lot better about the whole thing.

Another week or so into the roster and each shift has passed by uneventfully. We have fun, we perform as many interventions as we can, and we feel like our team is a force to be reckoned with. We enter our updated daily medication report en route back to the station. We don't need to check the bag itself for the vials. We just count up the medications from memory and the register that accompanies it. After dropping everything into the safe, we head home.

Just as we put our feet up, we receive a call from a manager, regarding a drug discrepancy and they ask us to come in early the next morning. As soon as we arrive, we realise that we have a fentanyl vial missing, but an extra, identical sized ampoule containing an anti-emetic is present.

As we rack our brains, we realise that there's a high likelihood of the vials having been mistaken. One of our patients must have been given an opioid rather than an anti-emetic. We will never know for sure whether this is the case, or, if so, which patient was administered the medication in error. Now that's the type of mistake to keep us awake at night. Wondering about the outcome for that patient, as well as the potential risk to our career.

No matter how much we justify not using the methods we were taught around safety checks and labelling, it remains almost impossible to find an acceptable argument against utilising tried and tested methods. This is a personal decision that we undertake, how stringent we are in our checks, but in precepting new staff, how can we possibly justify cajoling or forcing them into adopting our ugly habits? It took them long enough to learn how to do things the way they've been taught, persuading them to undo all of that hard work makes no sense for the patient, for themselves or their colleagues.

INFORMING THE INTERN -V- DODGING OUR DUTY

As we reach the end of the roster, we realise that we haven't completed any of the intern's on-road precepting paperwork. While colleagues have advised keeping it updated on a week-by-week basis, we didn't get around to it, so we sit down and start completing the forms. It turns out that there's a considerable amount to fill in and we're feeling frustrated by how long it's going to take. Realising that we won't be able to do it all on shift as it's too busy, we plan to take it home and complete it in our own time, even more frustrating as we have a lot to do on our days off already.

As soon as we settle into it, we calculate that it will be quicker just to tick the boxes. There's nothing outstandingly bad about the intern, so we don't want to cause them any problems and have them questioned about skill levels, therefore ticking them off as competent in everything saves us a great deal of time.

There are a couple of issues we don't particularly like about the intern's driving techniques, but we haven't bothered mentioning them because we didn't want to ruin the fun, friendly atmosphere in the ambulance. We're passionate about these areas, so we have to include them, otherwise they won't be rectified. We go on to outline the details for follow up by driver training staff.

Our partner is extremely quiet when we next see them at a nearby hospital. They look up as we enter, and quickly look away, no sign of the fun attitude they had when we were working together. Once our patient has been settled in a chair, we wander over and ask how they're doing.

"Fine." They reply and then turn away. A little confused, we ask if everything is okay, and they suggest that we step outside while their partner takes care of their sleeping patient. Only when they explain their shock at our written report, do we understand why this would be upsetting. They had thought everything was ticking along smoothly and had no idea that we had issues with their driving throughout the entire roster.

They inform us that had we mentioned it before, they could have rectified the situation. Only now, as it's currently written up in assessment documentation, the organisation have to act upon it, and the intern has been put back to the beginning of their driver training. An enormous setback to their career progression, their pay scale and their professional pride.

They ask us why we couldn't have mentioned it beforehand, but all we can fall back on is the excuse that we didn't want to ruin the fun atmosphere or friendly relationship. It sounds incredibly lame, even to ourselves.

We stepped up to this privileged position and realise that we have let our intern down badly when we should have been able to step up to the brave conversation. For the safety of the intern, patients and any colleagues who will be in the ambulance when they drive in future, all we had to do was speak up, but we took the easy way out and made it someone else's problem.

Communication and documentation are the only tools that preceptors are given to help a good paramedic forge ahead, or slow the progress of bad, or ugly, paramedic behaviours for the future. In most instances, any issues eventuating can be discussed with minimal discomfort immediately that they arise. The longer they are left, the harder they are to address. If they are not dealt with, they will develop and grow until they cause irreparable damage.

Ensuring right from the outset that nothing will be a surprise to the preceptee when our final paperwork is submitted will avoid potential discomfort in the first place. They soon become used to the idea that they'd rather hear feedback directly from us, the instant that it is recognised, than face formal follow up further down the track.

As long as we don't use ugly techniques to deliver the news, there's no need for the atmosphere to turn ugly. Openness, honesty and an awareness that it's part of our role as a preceptor in the first place help to swallow the bitter pill and get down to business. Otherwise, we risk losing our potential value in that role.

Why It Matters

Something often underestimated is just how impressionable a new paramedic, or intern, may be. This is not necessarily a personality trait, or specific to age, gender or background. It doesn't mean that the intern is easily led, or some kind of meek follower.

What it does mean, is simply that we have a new member of staff, who has worked incredibly hard to win this role and desperately wants to belong, within an industry renowned for its strength of character. Often, the easiest way to do so is to look around and see what other paramedics are doing. To fit in quickly and easily, the path of least resistance is most likely that of copying the majority.

The bulk of most interns' knowledge of ambulance world is gained from television, social media and hearsay, so the only other thing they have to go on, is what they see before them. If what they see before them are a majority that chooses to take shortcuts, it's immediately confrontational and challenging for them to go against that norm.

Were the majority to perform at the same standards they initially set for themselves upon entering the paramedic profession, however, it would be just as easy to create good paramedics from good students, with minimal effort required.

While most of us do maintain impeccable standards, on the whole, it's vital, when precepting, that we pay closer attention to how we let bad, or occasionally ugly, habits sneak into the picture.

We may find ourselves jumping in to take over during interventions before letting them try for themselves, causing our intern to miss out on opportunities and dulling their confidence in that area. Are we demonstrating safe and courteous emergency driving techniques, or do we give the impression that we own the road once the lights and sirens are on? Do we maintain sharps safety at all times? Are our clinical reports of a consistently high standard for patient and crew safety? If we have a habit of calling them "newbie" in front of patients and bystanders, are we making them feel exposed and vulnerable just for entertainment?

In most ambulance services worldwide, there is minimal training in precepting techniques. Often, all we have to go on is utilising the things we liked about our own preceptors and avoiding the things we didn't. We are regurgitating whatever we observed through our personal experience. With that in mind, there are some important considerations that we can use to keep ourselves accountable in this crucial role.

If we assume that every single intern will copy every single thing that we do on scene, are we going to be happy for them to attend our family members and mimic those behaviours?

Should we have the opportunity to observe our crew dynamic from the patient's perspective, are we seen in a supportive and encouraging role towards our partner for providing best patient care? Or are we creating any confusion, doubt or concern in the patient's mind?

Every time we disempower our intern with words, noises, gestures or facial expressions, their human instinct is to defend themselves against that happening again. The more we do it, the more defensive they will become. The more defensive they become, the more they will begin to disempower others using the same methods. The more they disempower any interns that they go on to precept, the more significant the cycle grows. Could this be the reason that new interns often appear arrogant and over-confident? Are they already on the defensive purely through the limited exposure they've had before their first shift?

Our good, bad and ugly habits spread like wildfire when we take on a precepting role. If each of us precepts only ten interns over the next few years, in less than two decades, those habits could replicate in over one million paramedics!

2020	1 preceptor influences x 10 interns = 10 potential new preceptors by 2023
2023	10 preceptors influence x 10 interns = 100 potential new preceptors by 2026
2026	100 preceptors influence x 10 interns = 1,000 potential new preceptors by 2029
2029	1,000 preceptors influence x 10 interns = 10,000 potential new preceptors by 2032
2032	10,000 preceptors influence x 10 interns = 100,000 potential new preceptors by 2035
2035	100,000 preceptors influence x 10 interns = 1,000,000 potential new preceptors by 2038

Avoiding honest feedback with interns about their performance creates a false sense of security, putting patients at risk, setting the intern up for a fall and ultimately, it may reflect upon us as a preceptor.

Refusing to request and hear feedback relating to individual precepting techniques, from interns, stops us from improving and prevents us from noticing when the bad and the ugly sneak in.

Failing to step up and document honestly is the quickest way to allow an ugly paramedic a free pass into the future. If we have an intern demonstrating a poor attitude, below-par skills, dangerous driving techniques and concerning levels of patient care at the early stages of their career, we cannot ignore it.

We are in a role whereby we are duty-bound to let that intern know our concerns as soon as they arise, document it thoroughly while the opportunity still exists and follow up with the body responsible for overseeing the intern's training.

Ultimately, we are growing paramedics for the future. Who is going to take care of us in our old age?

If we choose to avoid this responsibility and hope that another preceptor takes control of the situation, we may be sorely disappointed. That intern may become the paramedic that turns up at our own house to provide emergency medical assistance in the future.

Put Yourself In The Picture

Think back to your first preceptors or mentors. Who was fantastic, and why? Do you still use some of the habits you learned from them at the same high standard?

What about the other end of the scale, do you remember any awful experiences and whether you vowed at the time never to be that type of paramedic? Have you upheld that promise, or can you see the beginnings of some bad or ugly habits slipping into your practice?

If you're passionate enough about the paramedic role to deliver only the best to your interns, enjoy the thought of sharing your enthusiasm throughout the industry.

If you feel like you're losing the motivation to maintain the type of standards that you'd hope to see in one million future paramedics, you have a couple of options. Either liberate yourself from the preceptor role (if your ambulance service permits, please don't just quit your job) or speak to a trusted colleague about how to reignite your fire and energise the good paramedic habits that you'd love to share with future generations

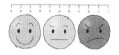

CHAPTER FIVE

DOCTORS, NURSES
& BRIDGING THE GAP

While the majority of paramedics build up friendly, respectful, professional relationships with the majority of nursing, medical and hospital staff, a certain level of animosity or rivalry appears to exist on a global scale. Evident in articles, textbooks, general conversation, social media and more.

Although attempts to explain the potential reasoning are often made, there exists a multitude of factors that may play a part. Experience, for all parties, is highly likely the major resounding factor that forms opinion early on, but this remains a two-way street.

Even though we may find that most hospital staff are professional, reasonable, work towards best patient care, and respond well to our handovers, we may occasionally experience a more difficult situation. The potential exists for that unpleasant feeling to overshadow all of the positive experiences leading up to it beforehand.

A common topic of conversation may be that of unpleasant interactions in the emergency department, and we all seem to have stories to add fuel to that fire, rather than focus on the countless positive experiences that counteract it.

From our point of view, we must represent our profession well, through our practices, so that nurses, doctors, patient care assistants and all other hospital personnel don't have their opinions of paramedics tainted by unnecessary bad or ugly behaviours.

The Good

To maintain good paramedic habits, it makes sense that our overarching concern remains that of best patient care. This helps us to form an easy to follow road map of how to behave while in the hospital domain.

It may involve smoothing the ripples arising in an awkward conversation. It may be necessary to stand firm in a specific area of patient advocacy.

More often than not, however, it merely requires us to maintain kind, professional and respectful human behaviour consistently.

PRE-NOTIFYING FOR PRIORITY -V- FAVOURING THE PHONE

We're en route to the local hospital with a polytrauma patient, after several hours of entrapment, in a high-speed motor vehicle collision. Our patient is sedated due to a suspected traumatic brain injury, has an apparent intra-abdominal bleed, along with a fractured pelvis and multiple smaller wounds to deal with.

Along with our partner, we've done a pretty good job of stabilising the patient, despite the extreme weather conditions and challenging multi-agency work involved in safe extrication. Now we have a police officer driving our vehicle so that we can both continue to treat en route.

As we dial the pre-notification number to provide an estimated time of arrival and case details, our patient's blood pressure drops again. We move forward in the vehicle to set up another bag of fluids while our partner is manually ventilating the patient through an endotracheal tube.

With the phone tucked under one ear, continuing to work, we calmly provide the bare essentials of the call and the patient's current condition, before stating how many minutes until we arrive, just as we're about to hang up.

The resuscitation team member at the other end of the phone, however, begins to ask for more specific details. We take a second longer to politely and firmly explain that we have no spare hands in the back of the ambulance, and need to attend to the patient urgently but will provide a full handover on arrival.

Although it's often frustrating to find ourselves in this situation during pre-notification, we have to remember how different our working environment is, to that at the other end of the phone.

To answer the call, the other party has stepped towards a telephone and, while their department may be overwhelmingly busy, their immediate focus at that moment is a notebook or whiteboard, upon which the details are scribbled as we speak.

They may have forgotten, or may not have ever seen, how a priority call looks in the back of an ambulance moving at speed. They may not understand that patient care is being undertaken in a confined space, by one or two, at best three paramedics, unrestrained in a moving vehicle.

From that person's perspective, therefore, it's in the patient's best interests that the receiving facility gains as much information as possible, in order to prepare the most suitable resources. Any refusal to provide details may appear obstructive or unreasonable on our part unless the paramedic can give some perspective from the patient's bedside.

By painting a quick picture of the limited resources we are working with, in a friendly manner, not only do we maintain positive interprofessional relationships, we form cohesive links in the chain of patient care.

SUPERVISING FOR SAFETY -V- HANDOVER HARM

Due to the limited information provided, the large trauma team assembled in the resuscitation bay are unsure of the patient's full injury status. They are keen to gain a more accurate picture. As we wheel the stretcher in, however, this immediately appears problematic, due to hands reaching out to remove monitoring equipment and safety belts, in an aim to speed up the transfer to the trauma bed.

We are aware that the risk to our patient, and all medical personnel, of something going wrong increases enormously at this point, because none of the movement is co-ordinated with any precision. With the patient still on our stretcher, we continue to wheel it forward, directly requesting that everyone leave the equipment and straps where they are for now so that our crew can safely remove them and be out of the way quicker.

The trauma registrar calls out for similar control, requesting that the patient be transferred when ready, and then for everyone present to tune in and listen to the paramedic handover.

This interprofessional collaboration is working beautifully in the patient's favour. Firm and clear instruction from ambulance personnel in maintaining safe control. Rather than an unco-ordinated "all hands on deck" approach. Similar firm and explicit instruction from hospital personnel, directing priorities to focus the team's efforts for rapid transfer.

Once we have removed the monitoring equipment, unfastened the safety belts, and carefully placed IV and IO lines out of harm's way, we push the stretcher up alongside the receiving bed. Our partner is still ventilating the patient, holding the tube in place, and they ask the receiving doctor to confirm its accurate placement before moving the patient across.

The airway registrar takes ten seconds to visualise the endotracheal device in situ at the vocal cords, before confirming, and a safe, smooth, slide transfer occurs. The stretcher is removed, providing a three hundred and sixty degree approach to the patient for the receiving resuscitation team.

We all know that it doesn't always work this way. Still, we can often steer it in this direction, if we maintain a patient-focused approach, rather than becoming frustrated or allowing ego to drive the situation. If we can be firm, direct and polite, with a focus on stating why the patient needs us to behave in a certain way, it helps to keep the recipients of our directive focused on the same goal.

Even on those occasions where an individual may appear to be unreasonable, or rude in their manner, all the while that we can maintain our focus, our professionalism is not under threat any more than our patient's safety is.

The risk lies, therein, when we become reactive to rude, or unreasonable behaviour and forget our focus. Not only do we then appear just as unprofessional as the instigator, but we also join them in jeopardising our patient's safety due to our complete shift in priorities.

KEEPING IT CONCISE -V- DISTRACTING WITH DETAILS

At this point, our partner wheels the stretcher out of the bay into a safe area of the corridor, allowing the hospital staff full use of the space available, and our handover begins. We pick a clear focal point, directing commentary towards the scribe, ensuring that they can both hear, and capture, all of the vital information relating to our patient.

By providing pertinent and specific details, with some volume, rather than quietly delivering a mix of information, we portray a high level of professionalism and clinical knowledge immediately. Where possible, we also aim to follow a recognised A to E or top to toe format. Rather than jumping from one bodily system to another and back again.

Further demonstrating that our clinical assessment and management follows the same, thorough, systematic approach.

In effect, if we garble a loose, difficult to follow handover, full of irrelevant information, we cannot help but be considered to operate in that way.

Our handover, documentation, and skill level evident in the interventions undertaken are the only means we have available to demonstrate our quality of clinical practice to staff in the hospital setting. Unless one of those doctors or nurses attends frequent shifts in the ambulance with us, their knowledge, opinion, and judgement will always have to be formed during only the brief periods in which we work together.

By consistently providing clear and direct pre-notification, attention to professional, clean, clinical interventions and packaging of the patient, along with well worded, easy to follow documentation and handover, we are automatically making it easy to regard us as efficient, well trained and educated professionals.

The Bad

Building our professional image is not a one-paramedic job. We can, individually, create a strong reputation for ourselves with nurses and doctors over time, the more we attend the same hospitals and work with the same staff towards the provision of medical care.

Overall, however, it's a team sport. No matter how hard we may work singlehandedly to demonstrate a high standard of patient care, medical knowledge and friendly approach, this can be undone in an instant by any one of us wearing the same paramedic uniform.

PROFESSIONAL PAUSE -V- UTTER ABANDON

We arrive one afternoon at our local emergency department and enter through the ambulance bay to find a nurse that we know relatively well, standing at the triage desk. After a brief chat, exchanging pleasantries between us, we begin our handover and explain what we've done for the patient prehospitally.

As soon as we enter, we notice that, in full view of the waiting room and all of the staff in triage, our partner leans against a wall then begins to scroll through their phone screen.

We glance up at them from time to time, hoping that they stop for a second and check on the patient or the monitor attached to the stretcher, but it doesn't happen. The nurse is entering our patient's details into the computer system at this point, and they, too, are beginning to look up at our partner. We start to feel uncomfortable.

We call out to our partner, asking them to check on the patient, but they simply look up at the stretcher and reply that they look fine. We walk over ourselves, observe the updated vitals on the monitor screen and reassure the patient that we'll be able to give them an update on what's happening once they are booked in.

Just as we're heading back to the triage desk, we notice a second nurse standing alongside, watching, who shakes their head and mumbles something about unprofessional paramedics, before disappearing.

There may be occasions where we have to take a phone call or send a message. We work for long periods without predetermined breaks or the ability to be contacted. We may often find, when we arrive at a hospital, that it's the first chance we get to check why our phone was vibrating with silent notifications during our last job. It's easy to deal with this openly and professionally, excusing ourselves briefly after explaining to our partner and ensuring that they, or another paramedic, are watching our patient and maintaining stretcher safety.

Perhaps our ambulance service provides protocols, guidelines and medication information via mobile apps, or we're looking up a medical condition after a discussion about how to give the best care for this patient between both crew members. Once again, all we have to do is outline our actions to the patient, our partner and anyone else concerned. Our body language in doing so will also differ from that of the switched-off paramedic, visibly leaning into their escapism, as they lean out of patient care mode.

From a hospital staff point of view, paramedics are quite possibly the only people involved in patient care who can be frequently observed using mobile phones at work. It's rare to see other medical personnel in a similar situation. There is possibly a sign nearby, requesting that mobile phones are not utilised, or even prohibiting them within that location.

While we're in a hospital, adhering to hospital policies and guiding our actions based on creating a professional impression, serves to maintain a professional image for ourselves as well as our paramedic colleagues.

DEFENDING OUR HONOUR -V- BURNING OUR BRIDGES

Later that day, upon returning with another patient, the nurse we'd heard muttering earlier is triaging all incoming ambulance cases. We've already written them off in our minds as harsh and unprofessional because it stung to listen to their comment when we were behaving professionally ourselves. It wasn't our fault that our partner acted the way they did.

The nurse looks up with a friendly smile and greeting, but we brush them off and jump straight into the handover. They look a little taken aback by our response but approach the business at hand in a similar detached manner, asking pertinent questions and ascertaining whether we have given any medications. We state that IV access was impossible. Therefore we've provided intranasal analgesia, and the nurse simply comments "Oh, of course."

We have no idea what this means, but we immediately assume that it's sarcasm. Relating to our inability to cannulate this patient, and our defensiveness increases.

The entire interaction has been tarnished by perception, on both sides. Although we feel justified in our judgement, that this nurse is harsh and unprofessional, because of their earlier comment, our behaviour only confirms that opinion.

In reality, her welcoming manner had provided us with the perfect opportunity to break down any misconception, but our ego may have jumped in and caused us to miss our chance. We cannot possibly know, or guess, how other health professionals perceive us, and it serves us no purpose in wondering. If we can simply behave in a pleasant manner, consistent with reasonable, professional expectation, we are representing ourselves, and our industry, at a good standard.

CLEARING THE AIR -V- RAMPING UP RESENTMENT

We have a little moment of indecision, during which the nurse looks at us, and we look at them, both wondering whether we should just say something. We consider the options and think about apologising, stating that we're not sure what has happened today, but we both seem to be butting heads, and perhaps could start over.

We're just about to start speaking when a patient collapses in the waiting room, and the moment is lost. By the time they return, we are standing by our patient, completing documentation and distracting ourselves from eye contact. No intention of revisiting that uncomfortable situation today.

Both parties have lost their focus on the patient, at the centre of shared care, and are instead attending more to our own defense. Both parties are unsure where they stand in the situation and what is happening. Both parties refuse to back down and openly address the issue. Both parties return to their respective colleagues and tell their perceived story about what happened. Both parties complain to their peers about the rude, disrespectful and unprofessional behaviour they just experienced.

In reality, comparing the two situations from an external perspective, not much actually happened.

A nurse made a disrespectful comment in passing, not ideal. A paramedic took offense and carried their frustration over to the next interaction, not ideal. The nurse was unclear in their communication regarding the cannulation comment. The paramedic assumed that the nurse was sarcastic, judgemental or rude. The nurse chose not to clear up any miscommunication, or let it go and start afresh next time, but instead chose to complain to others about paramedics. The paramedic chose not to clear up any miscommunication, or let it go and start afresh next time, but instead chose to complain to others about nurses.

This is how the gap between professions, in any industry, widens. If we don't take those golden opportunities to mention the elephant in the room, after awkward interactions such as this, it rarely comes up again in the future.

The nurse in question already had a poor opinion of paramedics, but was still open to friendly interaction, therefore susceptible to change that opinion if enough evidence to the contrary were presented. Rather than providing that evidence, through the exceptional standards we were attempting to demonstrate earlier in the day, despite our partner's behaviour, we simply supported their theory by being rude and dismissive.

No matter how difficult it seems, or how confrontational it may feel, best patient care dictates a necessity to discuss questionable action or inaction professionally and openly. Whether it is our own, or someone else's, the minute we remove any ego and focus on the need to prioritise both current and future patients' best interests, the conversation becomes so much easier.

Admittedly, it's not pleasant and, unless we lodge a litany of unnecessary complaints through our superiors to follow up, at management level between both organisations, there will be no-one else to do it for us. Some may see it as a downside to the autonomy in paramedicine. However, it's also part of the commitment we make to delivering the best patient care and maintaining our professional reputation.

Whether it's managing a scene, dispersing obstructive bystanders, removing fear by providing precise and direct instruction, increasing a patient's trust by explaining what's about to happen, or querying a negative interaction between caregivers. If we don't deal with it constructively, we leave an open space within which the situation may deteriorate, making it harder and harder to address every time it comes up.

Bad paramedic behaviour doesn't always have to be an active issue to lose the respect of other health professionals. Inaction is often just as damaging, perhaps more so in some instances.

Mutual respect is critical. If we disrespect other professions, by default, we can expect the same disrespect in return. If we wish to be respected, as an industry, we must earn it through consistent delivery of high professional standards, as well as maintain it through continued patient advocacy and standing firm upon our similar expectations of others.

The Ugly

As with many other areas of this book, the ugly section can be surprisingly unpleasant to read. What starts as small, occasional bad habits can unwittingly turn into ugly behaviours.

Sometimes we can't see it for ourselves. It has a way of sneaking up on us and infiltrating almost all of our clinical, professional and occasionally personal behaviours.

PRIORITISING PATIENTS -V- DEMONSTRATING DISREGARD

We're excited to be rostered permanently with a long-term colleague who has become a friend. We work the same way, have the same outlook on life, our manner with patients is the same, and we feel comfortable because they never challenge us unnecessarily.

As soon as our ambulance rolls up to the emergency department entrance with our patient, colleagues are calling out greetings and congratulations on the recent permanent partnership. We stroll in through the doors, our partner pushing the stretcher, and casually approach the triage desk, where we're asked if our patient is urgent, due to the growing queue building out in the waiting room. "Nah," we answer casually, "just an abdo pain."

As we lean down to the work surface, arms folded and start chatting to our partner and colleagues, we joke about how many patients we managed to walk into ED, rather than use the stretcher, on our last shift together.

Another paramedic asks our thoughts on the newly updated guidelines, released last week, and we laugh as we respond, in unison "What guidelines?" before declaring that we haven't bothered reading them yet. After almost twenty minutes, our patient calls out apologetically that they need to use the bathroom, somewhat embarrassed as they have to make themselves heard across a crowded triage area. We call back that they'll have to wait until we've been entered into the system and continue talking.

By this time, additional staff have been allocated to the busy department, allowing the original nurse to receive details regarding our patient now. They ask a few questions, with the same level of disinterest that we've demonstrated, complete the documentation while discussing an urgent issue with the ED consultant. They inform us that as our patient sounds currently stable and we have no concerns to mention, there will be a considerable wait. They joke that we'll be happy to carry on socialising for the time that we're ramped, and we laugh along with them.

The pleasant camaraderie we're experiencing feels easy, light-hearted and stress-free on a personal level. Still, its effect on our patient, as well as our professional reputation, can be insidious and ugly. From the moment we arrived and dismissed our patient's condition, the nurse took our word for it and didn't hesitate to prioritise a waiting room queue without further questioning.

Our patient, overhearing the interactions we're having, is uncomfortable, embarrassed and feeling insignificant as they wait, alone and without reassurance, in a crowded space, unwilling to press the issue of needing to use the bathroom.

While we don't need to rush the patient in and create unnecessary drama, it would be appropriate to explain that our patient has a gastrointestinal upset and we are happy to wait for initial triage but will let the nurse know if anything changes. Our patient's needs are validated, a high standard of patient care is maintained, and we remain adaptable to the busy hospital situation.

Emergency department staff may automatically maintain or increase respect for our role as clinicians, reducing the incidence of negative interactions as a result.

PROFESSIONAL POISE -V- EMBARRASSING INTERACTION

During our time spent waiting in the corridor, we wheel our patient to the bathroom, assist them back to the stretcher, then encourage them to sleep so that we can catch up with colleagues or watch a movie on our mobile devices.

There are several crews awaiting allocation to a bed, and the conversation turns to hilarity. Some patients are joining in with the chat, some are snoozing, but overall, the volume increases, the laughter intensifies, and the mood lightens further. A couple of paramedics stand quietly alongside their patients, chatting to them occasionally, checking vitals periodically and generally attempting to avoid the impending awkwardness.

When the nursing co-ordinator enters the corridor, looking irate, and requests that the noise be reduced, we're fully into the swing of things and call out for them to lighten up as they walk away. We've known them for years, and they're not usually so uptight, but there's no response, so we assume they haven't heard us.

A little later, however, a clerk arrives with some freshly printed posters and tapes them up on the corridor walls. The signs are marked for the attention of "ambulance drivers." Requesting that noise be kept to a minimum for the benefit of all patients within the department.

We are enraged. Some of our colleagues are enraged. We cannot believe that we are being treated so poorly, with such disrespect. Lengthy discussion ensues amongst some of the crews about the rivalry between nurses and paramedics. There is a suggestion of seeking management's support in submitting a complaint. Other paramedics remain silent and continue to maintain patient care just as they did before, now clearly embarrassed and frustrated by the situation.

Instances such as this are not isolated. A common observation by emergency department staff is that of watching or hearing, a group of paramedics behaving unprofessionally while ramped.

Even though we're standing, or occasionally seated, in a corridor, this does not eliminate our ongoing role in patient care. Despite the fact that we are now in a different working environment than our regular ambulance or on-scene surroundings, we remain responsible and accountable for the management and treatment of our patient.

If we behave like naughty children in this space, it's only natural that we will be treated as such.

Should we act in a manner likely to lose the respect of peer professionals, perhaps we have no cause for complaint in noticing that lack of respect. We cannot have it both ways. If we wish to be considered equals within the medical industry, we must act as equals at all times when in uniform and performing our role, no matter the circumstance.

For those who consistently work in favour of professional standards, it may be stressful, counterintuitive and extremely damaging for morale. To regularly face the difficult choice between speaking up and reminding colleagues to behave appropriately, as opposed to remaining silent and being judged negatively due to the behaviour of other paramedics, is punishing.

CONTINUITY OF CARE -V- INADVERTENT INATTENTION

Once our patient is allocated a bed, we wheel their stretcher through, but they do not stir. After calling their name and gently shaking their shoulders, the patient opens their eyes but appears quite sleepy.

It's only been an hour or so since our triage formally began and we spoke to them occasionally during that time, but after a brief handover, the receiving nurse asks what the last vitals were, due to the patient's altered conscious state. When we give the same numbers as the initial triage notes, they look up questioningly and ask when the observations were recorded. We admit, somewhat sheepishly, that they were last assessed in the ambulance before arriving, almost two hours ago.

We assist in the slide transfer from our stretcher to the hospital bed, noticing, at the same time as the nurse, that the patient has been incontinent on the stretcher. They had been wrapped up in blankets, so we had no idea.

The attending physician arrives and takes a quick look at the IV cannula in the patient's hand, which has become dislodged due to its loose tape. We hadn't noticed as the patient slept with their hands together under one side of their face for comfort, and we hadn't checked it at any time.

While the nurse is connecting the pulse oximeter, blood pressure cuff and three lead ECG, we notice that our patient is tachycardic. We start to feel a little unsettled about their condition, exchanging a glance with our partner. They clearly share the same concerns, as we wait for the monitoring equipment to register. The alarm sounds, our patient is hypotensive, and we are pushed out of the way as the bed is wheeled into the resuscitation bay urgently.

In paramedicine, it is common for there to be no strict rules in terms of monitoring a patient's vitals and condition when they are ramped. Many organisations request that this is in alignment with hospital policies, perhaps every half hour or so, but more often than not, it's at the paramedic crew's discretion.

In this type of scenario, at what stage are we considered negligent? If we forget or refuse, to continue care for a ramped patient, to the similar standard we felt was necessary before arriving in ED, we are letting them down badly. All the while that the patient remains on a paramedic crew's stretcher, in the care of that paramedic crew, we must uphold our obligation to best patient care and professionalism.

Every single time we, or our colleagues, demonstrate such low standards of care to nurses, doctors and other hospital staff, we cannot blame them for any poor opinion they may form of our profession.

No matter how many good paramedics demonstrate exemplary care, any cases of poor treatment will remain most memorable, ultimately tarnishing the reputation of every paramedic they represent.

Why It Matters

Crossing the divide between paramedics and other medical staff requires continuous and consistent effort. Despite the focus on hospitals within this chapter, this extends to other emergency service agencies, nursing homes, general practitioners, allied health professionals and more. The divide is bound to exist when we consider that, not so long ago, we were simply ambulance drivers. We drove to our patients, placed them in an ambulance, and transported them to the hospital so that other medical staff could assess and treat as necessary.

It's only in more recent times, and through gradual change, that we have developed such a broad-reaching skillset, which now ranges from ambulance driving, right through to advanced airway, surgical and pharmaceutical interventions. Like it or not, the benefit to our career progression in adding to our skills and knowledge, must be offset. A continual focus on proving that we are up to the task.

In many cases, a lack of education around the differences between our roles and work conditions prevents mutual understanding, and respect, from softening the edges as opinions are formed, removing judgement or resentment.

Without exposure to different working environments and skillsets, it's impossible to gain a real understanding of each other's roles. Therefore, it's essential to do our best to empathise with and educate from all points of view.

There also exists the problem created by additional demand for our adaptability. Many of us take great pride in the dynamic attitude required to continually work within any and every type of environment imaginable, purely due to the unknown nature and location of every single call we attend. An element of the bluff helps us to manage this challenge admirably. Still, after most calls, it also falls to us to leave behind that bluff, forget the autonomy temporarily and play by the hospital's rules.

For some, this may feel like torture. The lack of fresh air, freedom and autonomy may seem almost debilitating, but it's an inevitable part of the role, without the potential for change in the near future.

For others, however, this may be a time of relief from relentless ambulance calls. A period during which the environment is more predictable, the rules of patient care are well defined, support exists in managing complex patient needs or threats to our physical safety, and we have access to luxuries such as bathrooms and coffee! All we have to do is maintain regular vitals and continued quality of care of our patient.

If it proved necessary to provide analgesia, fluids, cardiac monitoring and other interventions en route, an adequate continuation of care will more than likely require the same while ramped. Either upon arrival or if the successful treatment effects diminish.

Should the patient's condition not have improved significantly before arriving, there is no justification in ceasing that treatment simply because we're now inside a hospital building instead of an ambulance. Ideally, suitable ongoing medication may be arranged in collaboration with emergency department staff. If not, it seems outrageous that the same level of care delivered en route would stop just because our patient is in limbo between the ambulance and a hospital bed.

Conversely, our patient may be feeling more comfortable as a result of the treatment provided and wants to sleep. These occasions are great opportunities to catch up on reading journal articles, researching medical questions arising from previous jobs or other work-related tasks.

This may be considered perfectly reasonable within most ambulance services, as long as it is handled professionally and thoughtfully. Outlining a plan to our patient, that we will be catching up on mobile device based work, but will still be right with them, keeps the change in dynamic open and upfront.

We can still wake them to check on their condition periodically and set ourselves up for either automatic acquisition or manual reassessment of vitals at regular intervals. Such a combination permits the best use of time, best patient care and a high level of ongoing professionalism.

Remember that although this book is for paramedics, it does not mean that such behaviours or habits are limited to our profession. Bad apples are bad apples. Just like paramedics, there are plenty of good, bad and ugly examples of hospital staff, which we simply cannot avoid from time to time.

We will all have experienced demonstrations of poor practice, frustrating interactions, or unprofessional behaviour towards ourselves, and our patients. These negative experiences may rapidly distort our perception of entire professional groups, rather than assigning them to the individual responsible. In the same way that each paramedic hopes that they are not judged solely on their colleagues' behaviours, we must hope that we don't judge others only on the actions of their peers.

The human factors involved in negotiating the fine line between consistent patient advocacy, professionalism and teamwork with other health professionals are complicated and innumerable. If we could remove those factors, it would more than likely lead to a straightforward, unemotional and efficient, patient-centred transaction.

Fortunately for us all, however, there are no apparent moves towards replacing medical staff with robots. Otherwise, this type of transaction would also involve us losing the friendships, camaraderie and countless happy, rewarding moments we gain from our interactions over the years.

For patients, it's those same human factors that result in the excellent examples of outstanding, empathetic care they desperately need, just as much as the clinical treatment they receive.

No matter how much effort we put into maintaining high standards of clinical skill, patient care and interprofessional relationship building, the overall reputation of prehospital professionalism depends on the next paramedic to walk through each hospital's doors. If we undo the ugly, break the bad and grow the good habits in our profession, only then can we expect to gain full recognition and unwavering respect.

Put Yourself In The Picture

How do you perform when you're under the spotlight in your local hospitals? Do you have a reputation as a good clinical operator, or are you well known for clowning around when ramped?

If you felt a little awkward about your behaviour reading this, it's never too late to make a change. Maybe it will be easier for others around you to do the same, and they were just waiting for someone else to lead the way.

Are you often embarrassed by colleagues or do you feel that as a group, the majority represent our profession well? Perhaps it's worth mentioning your thoughts in either case. Speak up if a paramedic is behaving poorly, but just as importantly, acknowledge the aspects that you're proud of, giving others the chance to feel proud of their professionalism too.

How about the difficult interactions with other health professionals? Do you find yourself voicing your concerns if a doctor, nurse or another member of hospital staff passes comment, or behaves as if you've done something unacceptable? Or do you prefer just to let it go and avoid the hassle?

Consider setting yourself some rules. For example, if it's going to affect patient care or damage your reputation, maybe you'll request a moment for private conversation and address the issue. If it's only your pride that's being affected, perhaps you'll ignore it. Forming clear benchmarks and pathways for yourself, in advance, may take the stress out of the situation when it arises in future.

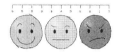

CHAPTER SIX

LEADERSHIP
IN THE SPOTLIGHT

In every example covered in earlier chapters, we have a work partner. Good, bad, or ugly, we have a crew mate by our side. No matter whom we work with, or how we've worked in the past, once we step out of that double crew dynamic, everything changes.

We no longer have a buffer to keep us on the straight and narrow through the good practices they model. Gone are the bad habits we see in some partners as reminders of what not to do. While we may have escaped the exposure to ugly behaviours that some colleagues have subjected us to, we only have ourselves to rely upon now, and the spotlight intensifies on everything we do.

Any opinion that we've mentioned to colleagues regarding organisational management in the past, from clinical decisions through to what we'd change if we could, now helps to form their new expectations of us. Anything that we criticised in conversation about single responders, managers and leaders, will be recalled when we show the slightest hint of heading down that same path.

Throughout this chapter, we can think of the ambulance service as a pyramid, by way of illustrating the shape of its most common leadership structure. Although not all ambulance services are structured in the same way, the resounding factor that does not change is that without patients, there is no ambulance service.

Without paramedics, those patients cannot receive the product that an ambulance service is designed to provide. Without support roles, those paramedics cannot receive the information, communications, dispatching, equipment, vehicles, medications, technology, training, infrastructure and more that they need to provide that product. Without managers, these support roles and paramedic roles cannot be organised effectively to streamline product delivery. Without leaders, these managers cannot specify the direction required to ensure that patients receive the highest quality of product possible from the ambulance service they've called.

The ultimate role of every single individual within the organisation exists to provide care to patients.

If we look at this pyramid, populated by paramedics providing frontline care at its base, we can then look at managerial and leadership roles further up on the scale. This approach in no way represents any suggestion of varying importance, or that one is "higher up" or "above" any other. What it means is that we have a clear way of understanding to whom we directly provide our services, from whichever position we may currently hold.

As a single responder, manager, or leader, we have chosen to step into our leadership role for some reason that has particular meaning to us. In doing so, we have opted to step up and deliver added value to those in our care, therefore the expectation now upon us to do so, is fair, reasonable and entirely justified.

The Good

Bringing pre-existing, long term good habits, into leadership roles will undoubtedly make the difference between having to work hard to earn respect in our new capacity, and automatically being considered worthy of the increased responsibility and benefits our new position entails.

Through this good reputation, not only do we immediately promote high standards by example, but we also create opportunities to encourage positive conversation and maintain enthusiasm in those paramedics who invariably aim for best practice.

SERVING THE SOLE PURPOSE -V- LOSING THE WAY

It's going to be a busy day, our schedule is full of tasks to complete, along with a couple of meetings, and we're under pressure to catch up with several paramedics at the request of senior management. Just as we walk away from our desk to get started, however, the phone rings and a local crew request assistance with an equipment issue. They are on scene with a severely unwell bariatric patient, but the lifting cushion has failed, and despite talking them through steps that often rectify the situation, we cannot solve the problem. Specialist technical support will be required.

After arranging for backup assistance in the short term, we inform the crew by phone that while they take care of the patient, we will find out what needs to happen. We contact technical support, book the lifting equipment in for review, then arrange for a replacement to be swapped into the ambulance as soon as possible. At this point, we email the crew to inform them. As well as provide a link to the reporting system so that they can complete the necessary paperwork as soon as their patient has been handed over.

Although we no longer spend as much time, if any, in face-to-face contact with emergency callers, every ambulance role is designed to facilitate the highest volume and quality of patient care available. It may be quicker to call the paramedic and let them know how they can resolve the issue. Still, all this will do, is save our own time, immediately prioritising our precious minutes above that of the ambulance crew.

On occasion, it's also essential for us to provide written evidence of our interactions, particularly if it has impacted directly upon patient care in some way. Whether it's pharmacological advice by phone, hands-on clinical intervention on scene, or technical assistance relating to equipment, if we expect the attending paramedic to document such information, we must provide them with similar text regarding our part in the proceedings. Our familiarity with phrases such as "If it isn't documented, it didn't happen" applies no matter which position we hold.

In this instance, although we may have spent extra time in facilitating a solution and documentation, how much time have we freed up for frontline patient care? The crew may now save our email for future reference or copy and paste the details of our part in the interaction, if necessary, into the patient report form.

They won't waste time chasing up equipment and can easily click on the link to reach the reporting form that must be completed, saving us from having to follow up at a later date. Our part in the proceedings is neatly tied up, we can move on to other tasks, the crew will be ready for their next call in less time, and the organisation has more paramedics available to meet patient demand.

FULLY INFORMED -V- DANGEROUS ASSUMPTION

As soon as we manage to leave our office and become mobile for the day, we are called to a significant trauma case to provide clinical assistance. From the second we arrive, it's evident that the scene is noisy, chaotic and crowded with onlookers. We notice the initial attending crew dealing with a patient and intuitively gravitate towards an elderly couple, crying inconsolably, with several bystanders reassuring them.

Rather than stop, we quickly check if there are any other patients, and assure them that we'll be right back, as soon as we've touched base with the other paramedics on scene. We manage to convey a sense of calm and control within seconds, by keeping this small group informed, while also taking the opportunity to glance over them and ascertain that none have any immediately obvious life-threatening issues.

After asking the crew how we can help and hearing their brief handover regarding the patient's vitals and mechanism of injury, we immediately take action in providing the best support possible. We call for urgent backup and work alongside them until assistance arrives.

As soon as the second ambulance shows up, we're now free to either allocate resources to the second patient or tend to them ourselves, as well as ascertain the full extent of their injuries and ensure that there are no other casualties nearby. Had we not prioritised initial handover of information, we may have compromised patient care and crew safety in favour of treating a low acuity patient.

As a single responder, when we are called for additional support, the good paramedic can maintain that level of care, to both crews and patients. As paramedics, we implore receiving medical facility staff to focus objectively on the information and findings we have obtained from the scene, rather than form a subjective opinion of what they see before them after the fact. Similarly, we must provide that same objectivity upon our arrival. It may appear obvious to us, in terms of what needs to be prioritised, but unless we are first on scene, we may not have all of the information available.

In regular paramedic roles, when we arrive to provide backup, the good paramedic tends to defer to the attending clinician upon arrival, rather than automatically taking over. At a major incident, the commanding officer gains pertinent information as a matter of priority before initiating further action. In our leadership roles, the same rules apply.

If we don't know what actually happened, then we can't know what potential dangers exist. If we are unsure of what the paramedics on scene are dealing with, then we cannot be sure of what our priorities are. If we aren't clear about which resources are required to manage the scene adequately, then we will fail to organise the appropriate resources.

For our safety as well as that of the patient and other emergency personnel, we absolutely must prioritise gaining some type of handover, no matter how senior our role.

TREAT & RUN -V- ADDING VALUE ON SCENE

With the initial crew departing for the trauma centre under lights and sirens, we shift our attention to the elderly patients and bystanders awaiting assistance. As the backup team begin to ascertain their injuries, the husband and wife couple tell us that they don't want to go to hospital, indicating minor scratches to their hands as the only damage sustained.

We suggest that between the three of us, we can fully assess both patients, complete their patient care records and refusal documentation, as well as clean up our mess at the scene and prepare their ambulance for the next call. We call control and notify them that we're available for backup and assistance, should an urgent call come in, but in the meantime, we utilise the time to work with our colleagues in getting the job done.

Some of the most valuable opportunities for debriefing, rapport building and gaining insight into current areas of satisfaction, or discontent, arise from merely working together. Not only is this useful from a managerial point of view, it's also precious for our colleagues, and ourselves.

Frustration around single responders turning up on high acuity jobs, getting stuck into the intensive work, then disappearing before transportation, clean up and paperwork begins, is common in the prehospital environment.

Distance and loss of connection between frontline employees and managers or leaders rapidly occur as soon as we lose the chance to converse naturally over shared tasks. Resentment grows rampant amongst those who feel that they're doing the hard work while others step in and "take the glory."

Realistically, this level of teamwork is not always possible in a single responder or leadership role. We may be continuously caught up in meetings and administrative tasks. There may be such a high number of calls that the "treat and run" approach is unavoidable. Merely acknowledging it makes a huge difference, however.

The good paramedic can easily find a balance, through acknowledgment and action. A pattern of bad habits may lead us to swoop in full of self-importance, treat and run, without actually acknowledging the crew on scene and potentially unsettle, frustrate and de-rail what had been running smoothly before our arrival.

Alternatively, through maintaining good habits, in the same amount of time, we may arrive, gain a handover and ascertain what the crew needs assistance with, before providing the treatment, support or interventions required.

Such an inclusive approach garners trust, reassures the paramedics on scene that we are not seeking "glory" or an opportunity to take over. With this ongoing, regular behaviour, when we are under pressure to respond to multiple calls, the good paramedic acknowledges the situation. We can still exit the scene rapidly, but at the same time, we apologise that we have to rush off to another tasking and thank the crew for taking care of the rest of the job.

Next time we catch up with them, simply helping to clean a stretcher, re-stock equipment or make a cup of coffee continues to demonstrate our view that we're all working together towards best patient care.

Our managerial, leadership or support roles are designed around frontline paramedics. We expect them to aim for best patient care, therefore, as individuals, and as an organisation, we must manage, lead or support them in their endeavours.

The good paramedic in this space comes to the fore when we continually maintain such focus. As soon as we turn the pyramid upside down, and begin to prioritise our role, our time or our needs, we no longer add the value that our frontline colleagues justifiably expect to see.

The Bad

With the upward trajectory of any promotional role, the pyramidal structure naturally exposes us to closer scrutiny. In an ambulance service, the structure is bottom-heavy with frontline paramedics, amongst others, into which good, bad and ugly behaviours are easily absorbed and can go relatively unnoticed for some time.

Once we step up out of that crowded space, we are no longer surrounded by so many of our peers. Therefore our performance is observed more closely. The pressure increases upon us to support, impress and appease both the colleagues we used to be surrounded by, as well as the line managers and leaders to whom we are directly accountable.

Not only does this apply to the individual in this realm, but management and leadership as a whole. Any display of bad habits and poorly managed situations at this level is no longer limited to a patient versus paramedic sized arena. It may now be broadly analysed and discussed to such a degree that distrust and disappointment quickly begin to run amok amongst the entire paramedic workforce.

CLEAR BENCHMARKS -V- MOVING TARGETS

After a recent promotion, we're keen to make a positive impression and begin by setting ourselves the target of completing several scheduled performance reviews before the day is out. Having approached our line manager for a review template to work from, we are directed to a loosely based list of questions, with little emphasis on creating a direction for future focus and minimal benchmarking capability. We're steadily working through them, using our own additional questions to provide more structure, when we sit down to work through an appraisal with a paramedic whom we've never met.

We are surprised by their lack of concern when we raise an issue that is documented as having been problematic in previous years. We mention that they don't seem too concerned by the matter, and they explain that our predecessor had dismissed it as unimportant in the past; therefore, they didn't think it would come up again.

Upon further discussion, we are dismayed to hear that their previous manager had utilised a different structure, similarly based around the loose proforma provided by the organisation, but with a different focus. We're frustrated and disappointed that we're attempting to offer a structured approach to the performance reviews, only to find that other managers, past and present, have also formed their own methods, creating inconsistent appraisal tools.

As a leadership group, therefore, we realise that we're placing all staff in an impossible situation. Without clear expectations, benchmarks and objectives, we can't possibly expect them to know what they're aiming for. We arrange an urgent appointment with our manager in an attempt to rectify the situation as soon as possible.

The next morning, we take our documentation and concerns into the meeting, only to be told that this subject has been raised before, and the proforma template is simply for guidance only. Our line manager states that it's up to the individual to go through the process and make their assessment on whether each paramedic is meeting the organisation's standards or not. "This is the way it has always been done." Although some peers reported problems with it initially, they all found ways of working around it; therefore, it shouldn't be an ongoing issue.

We're horrified to realise that this is one of the problems that often came up on road, in our paramedic role. On so many occasions, we have heard others discussing the ambiguity around the review process, and now we are experiencing it firsthand.

From an ambulance service point of view, this lack of consistency may cause so much confusion and frustration, in unsuccessfully reaching for unattainable, invisible or unknown targets, that many good paramedics gradually stop caring.

No matter how hard both parties involved in a review or audit situation try to make it work unless each remains consistent in their approach, there can be no way of setting standards and no way of measuring them accurately. If we can set specific and clearly defined goals, in alignment with specific and clearly defined criteria, we may find that the natural paramedic desire to meet, and exceed expectations, lends itself seamlessly to successful outcomes time and time again.

Once we lose the active participation of either party, the process loses its value, and distrust on both sides looms larger.

As a manager, we now find ourselves in the first of perhaps many situations that begin to test our good, bad and ugly approach in a different realm. Do we accept the feedback we've been given and continue to adapt the review to suit our standards? This may be the easiest way, and we don't want to make waves this early in our new role. Or do we take the stance that someone has to attempt to rectify the situation?

We decide to sleep on our moral dilemma but remain painfully aware of the relative increase in benefit, or potential damage. Any action, or inaction on our part, rather than affecting just one patient, may now affect a large number of frontline paramedics employed, and ultimately the patients they attend to in the future.

ACKNOWLEDGING THE GOOD -V- REWARDING THE BAD

After thinking it over, we plan to re-visit the issue in a couple of weeks and see how we feel about it then, allowing us to leave it on the backburner while we tackle the long list of performance reviews outstanding. The remaining number is easier to work through as we've become more familiar with our own method of appraisal, and we enjoy the opportunity to sit down with so many paramedics, going over past, present and future performance goals and outcomes.

Upon completion, our compiled report reveals large numbers of staff that are continuously working hard with a future-focused approach. They appear to be maintaining excellent levels of patient care, documentation and work ethic, with healthy goals for the upcoming year.

A small number of bad, and a few ugly paramedic habits have been highlighted through this process, and we're about to present them to the review board. We're also pleasantly surprised to note that two paramedics, usually renowned for their poor practices and unacceptable behaviours, seem to be turning things around in a positive direction.

The overall tone of the meeting is excellent, our peers, line managers and senior leadership team are also glad to see the results of our review, along with similar findings from others. As a group, we plan how to manage the potentially problematic side of things before any issues arise. An email is drafted for distribution to all paramedic staff, highlighting the bad and ugly practices in question, providing a reminder of the risks involved and the importance of avoiding them.

It is also decided that a manager will go and congratulate the two paramedics making positive change, to acknowledge their efforts verbally and enthuse others.

From the ambulance service's position, these steps may appear necessary, proactive and helpful in aiming for best practice across the board. The adverse reaction that ensues, therefore, is an unpleasant shock when it filters up from the frontline, through team leaders and departmental line managers.

It would appear that the majority of paramedics are frustrated and angry. The steadfast and reliable majority, with their consistently good habits and behaviours, feel that they are continually ignored, and now view the email as an insult. The general mood appears to be around feeling "tarred with the same brush" by the decision to remind good paramedics that the minority bad, or ugly behaviours are unacceptable.

Adding insult to injury, the focus on rewarding those suddenly aiming to do the right thing, when others who have always done so, feel that they are never acknowledged for it. An extremely sensitive area and often a "no man's land" type of situation, as both groups may struggle to understand the other's point of view.

Leadership groups generally know what they expect from frontline staff, that they show up for work and provide the service as agreed upon accepting their position. The reward is that of being paid. Expecting a "pat on the back" for doing their job may be considered unreasonable.

If a pattern emerges around bad or ugly behaviours, notification of this seems proactive, surely, in providing direction around what will not be tolerated. As far as the employees who have taken steps to improve their work practices are concerned, doesn't it make sense that we acknowledge and congratulate those efforts so that they continue on that path?

The majority of frontline staff, however, may not necessarily know what a leadership group's expectations are. They no doubt agree that showing up for work, providing excellent service and being rewarded through regular payment is reasonable. The confusion, therefore, often arises as a result of each organisation's approach, and the cultural tone it sets. For example, whether it appears reactive and based on negative behaviours, or proactive, based on the positive, thereby demanding positive practice as an ongoing standard.

In a reactive ambulance service, unclear expectations and shifting benchmarks make it difficult for everyone, at every level, to stay on track. Without a clear definition of desirable goals, there is no defined path to follow on a day-by-day basis. Such lack of clarity around what is considered unacceptable makes it impossible to know what to avoid. Any inconsistency in deterrent, ranging between discouragement and punitive action, makes it easier for the bad and ugly to test the boundaries. Without regular updates regarding performance, the majority will have no idea whether they're on track or not. Reactively stumbling around, as a fragmented organisation, automatically defines a "them" and "us" situation, purely by way of self-preservation against the fear of the unknown.

In a proactive ambulance service, however, support and encouragement towards maintaining good practice must be the focus. Setting clear expectations around what is acceptable and desirable provides easy to follow direction. Clarity around what is considered unacceptable provides the vision required to know what must be prevented. Consistent punitive action demonstrates clearly that boundaries are firm, helping to avoid bad and ugly behaviours insidiously creeping in as part of the unofficially accepted culture. Regular and reliable contact to provide feedback on how the majority is performing keeps the general direction on track. Proactively aiming together, as a team, towards a shared goal, automatically reduces the potential divide between "them" and "us" through shared ownership of the task at hand.

While this approach is unrealistically simplified into two basic paragraphs, for the sake of easy reading, it is in no way an easy undertaking.

Proactivity, and sticking consistently to a robust and overriding focus, however, may be the deciding factor in ensuring success or failure. Each time a leadership team makes any decision, or change, or needs to provide clarity around a specific topic, clear communication regarding why, what we're aiming for, and when we'll be checking in, may demonstrate clear expectations and accountability. Consistent follow up at the promised check-in time, regarding the success, failure and future direction of each issue, may promote ownership and increase trust.

Reliably following a consistent, replicable and recognisable method of communication may ultimately serve as the central, strong backbone in supporting an organisation. If the majority are excited by the prospect of a particular change, it becomes vital to consistently keep everyone in the loop, to maintain that interest and ensure its success.

Should an area of confusion or repeat questions arise, addressing the issue, through this method, assures the majority that their concerns are acknowledged, and demonstrates the proactive nature of the organisation by communicating in this way. Even if the majority are likely to disagree with a policy, or it may cause unrest and upset, maintaining this level of contact demonstrates that it's non-negotiable, and may make it easier for frontline paramedics to accept and promote its success.

OWNING WEAKNESSES -V- BLUFFING STRENGTHS

After dealing with the backlash of this inflammatory email all day, we are tasked to a multi-casualty incident, involving dozens of patients at a nearby sports ground. We receive a phone call en route, advising us of the updated SITREP, relayed by the crews on scene. When we arrive, a paramedic is standing at the entrance, attempting to direct us to park in a specific area.

We ignore them, however, as we have been tasked to co-ordinate the scene, and enter the grounds, leaving our vehicle as close as possible to the gates. We don our incident commander vest and walk towards the growing crowd of walking wounded and bystanders, noticing a paramedic who seems to be pointing people in different directions.

We ask for an update and are given precise details of the incident, the number of casualties and the resources involved, before informing the paramedic that they can begin treating a patient in their ambulance. The paramedic appears quite shocked and suggests that perhaps we should continue to work through the sieve and sort process of triaging, as well as finalise the setup of a casualty clearing post, treatment zone and so on. Still, we advise that we'll be able to take care of that so that they can focus on their clinical role.

As soon as the paramedic leaves, we take out our major incident pocket guide and realise our mistake. We didn't pay attention to the scene on arrival, and not only ignored the attempt to direct us toward an ambulance assembly area, but we have parked our vehicle inappropriately; therefore it will have to be moved. We refused to listen to the paramedic already in control, using our bluff to try and convey a sense of authority and missed the opportunity to recognise that they were clearly well versed in managing such a scene. We failed to prepare ourselves for this part of the role upon receiving our promotion.

These moments of realisation are a compelling teacher. Particularly for a single responder, manager or leader in the spotlight. Away from the comfort of the crowd of paramedics that we're used to blending in with. If we are stepping up into a role, we absolutely must know exactly what that role entails. If we are expected to provide clinical advice, and we come up against something we're not sure about, we absolutely must be willing to either provide reliable information or drop our bluff, admit that we don't know and defer to other sources that do.

Should our role entail being tasked to manage mass casualty calls, we must ensure that we know how to follow internationally recognised major incident plans. If we have any doubt, we absolutely must be willing to drop the bluff and utilise the experience of those around us to manage it most effectively.

This transitional period may prove incredibly challenging for many paramedics. The very nature of the role that we are most comfortable in is that of getting things done, fixing things up and dealing with situations that we are unexpectedly thrown into. While our bluff may have been useful and protective in such instances, once we're operating at managerial, support or leadership levels, hiding behind it may place patients, staff and interagency personnel in danger.

Every time we refuse to accept that we need help, or don't know an answer to something, two extremely damaging outcomes have the potential to occur. Our cover may be blown, and those around us realise that we are bluffing. As a result, we may lose credibility, respect and trust in the eyes of our fellow professionals; therefore, it's unfair of us to expect them to trust our role in the future.

More devastating, however, is that our bluff remains intact, our pride undamaged, but someone gets hurt. Either a patient is harmed by our refusal to acknowledge that we were unsure, or colleagues are injured because we fumbled our way through a procedure and missed a vital point designed to protect first responders.

Bad paramedic behaviours, at a leadership level, involve bigger, badder repercussions. If we make efforts to understand our responsibilities fully, we can then see where any gaps in our knowledge lie, providing us with the opportunity to fill those gaps before they cause a problem.

If we can drop the bluff and acknowledge our weaker points, with transparency and humility, we create more trust in those around us. If leadership groups ensure that specific roles are filled with specially trained staff, we can more easily ensure optimal safety for patients, employees and any others who may be affected by the decision-makers involved.

The Ugly

As with any paramedic role, noticing a trend in our behaviours, towards ugly practices, is a learned art.

At any leadership level, it is even more critical that we become highly skilled in doing so, through self-reflection, seeking feedback and actively listening to the information provided.

If we continue to work on the premise that a more visible role is scrutinised, and judged, more profoundly, it stands to reason that any ugly behaviour runs the risk of immediately undermining all of the good that we may previously have demonstrated up until that point.

ASSIGNING IMPORTANCE -V- DISMISSING CONCERN

After progressing through various clinical and managerial leadership roles, we now find ourselves settled into the senior management team. We've noticed that our day-to-day concerns have begun to change. The items that we have to focus on have become less frontline in nature. Less paramedic focused and more closely related to aspects of the organisation that we didn't even realise existed until now. It's a steep learning curve, but we're managing the change well, and feedback on our performance is positive.

Today's primary focus is our annual state conference; therefore, we have a presentation to prepare for, as well as ongoing liaison with our team around various current issues, so it's a high-pressure day. Mid-way through the morning, our phone rings and we are surprised to hear the voice of an old paramedic colleague, still working on road, whom we haven't seen for a long time. After exchanging pleasantries, they tell us that they're calling because they're not sure who else to turn to for assistance.

The matter is related to a new item of ambulance equipment. The paramedic has complained to several managers about the potential it has to cause hand injuries, but without success. They explain that they have followed our service's procedures, drafted a business case for change, backed it up with evidence-based findings regarding the likelihood of harm and still haven't been taken seriously.

While on the phone, we become distracted by the arrival of an urgent email and feel pressured by time as we realise that we only have an hour left before an important meeting. The caller asks if we have heard what they've said, and despite reassurance that we're listening, the very fact that they had to ask, tells us that they know our attention is elsewhere.

It's slightly frustrating, we're doing our best to give them our time, but we're also under a lot of pressure, and we know that this particular piece of equipment was the most cost-effective option for the organisation. We explain that we are swamped, but promise to look into the situation and get back to them.

They go on to explain that their work partner was almost injured this morning, that's why they're escalating the matter now before someone gets hurt, but we're at a loss to know how we can help. We have a relationship with this paramedic, we worked together for several years, so in our discomfort, we fall back on our usual humour. As we make a joke about the number of incident reports that paramedics love to lodge, in an attempt to lighten the mood, we notice that it doesn't go down well. They sound disappointed, and despite our efforts to rectify the situation with an assurance that we'll be in touch, they hang up, clearly disheartened.

In this instance, we realise that we have failed those whom we are tasked to look after. Just as the paramedic role is to provide the best patient care, our position, in leadership, is to provide the best paramedic care. We have turned the pyramid upside down by forgetting our purpose and viewing our role as more important.

We must take any concern seriously, as soon as it is brought to our attention. We may find it trivial or inconsequential at whichever level we're currently working within our organisation. To the person raising the issue, however, they have more than likely ruminated on the problem for some time before bringing it to anyone's attention. It may not be our immediate priority, but as our role is designed to support paramedics in providing the care that keeps our organisation in existence if a problem is raised, it must be added to our list.

Any attempt to dismiss such concerns, just because they are not affecting our own day to day function, harms our reputation. Be it seriously intended, or even good-humoured, discouragement of lodging safety or incident reports, because it creates more work for us, demonstrates that we prioritise our own time more highly. Presuming to know another employee's role, despite having stepped out of it several years ago, indicates our refusal to acknowledge that we may be out of touch.

Whether we deal with the actual problem ourselves or direct it to the most appropriate party for follow up, we rely upon frontline staff to highlight any concerns. The minute they stop caring, just because we've stopped caring, the whole organisation is at risk.

SUPPORTING STAFF -V- FITTING IN WITH FRIENDS

After hanging up, we get back to the increasingly pressing matters that were building and do our best to get through as much work as possible before rushing off to our scheduled meeting. The meeting runs smoothly, our presentation is well received, and our busy week culminates in the cocktail bar after the conference ends.

It's such a great atmosphere, not only do we enjoy a couple of drinks with the leadership team, line managers and support staff, but we get to catch up with several paramedics whom we haven't seen for years.

We're engrossed in conversation with a partner from way back, when the rest of their group decide to head out to a local club and catch up informally, away from the work arena. Still chatting intently with our colleague, we travel with them and spend the evening laughing, drinking, dancing and reminiscing about old times.

We meet several new paramedics and get to know them over drinks, some commenting with surprise that we're "out with the troops", but we hit the tequila with them and prove that nothing's changed just because of our role. We pose for photos with the rest of the group, raising our glasses, laughing, arms around each other. At the end of the night, we catch a cab home, feeling inebriated but happy and connected through that old camaraderie that never really leaves.

After a great sleep and a relaxing weekend, Monday comes around, and we arrive back in the office to a barrage of emails piling up in our inbox. We scan through them and find that one of the paramedics at the nightclub has posted inappropriate photos of themselves on a couple of social networking sites, which have been flagged by our media team. The paramedic in question isn't someone we know well, but we met them briefly on Friday night, and we're informed that they have received warnings about this in the past due its contravention of our organisation's social media policy. We are scheduled to attend a meeting first thing this morning, with the paramedic, their industrial representative and human resources.

We only need imagine the horror in chairing this meeting. In our professional, leadership capacity, which we stepped into by choice, we are now expected to facilitate disciplinary proceedings. The details swim around in our conscience. We hung out with them on the night in question, drinking alcohol, partying together. It is highly likely that we will feature in some of the photos to be used in the proceedings.

We forged a personal relationship with them and shared jokes about work-related stories. The situation feels impossible. Not only are we feeling the discomfort at the thought of answering questions from leadership team colleagues and directors, but we feel terrible for the paramedic. Just as we're terminating their employment, we can't help but ask ourselves how ugly our part in the proceedings may appear.

Becoming a leader in paramedicine does not mean that we have to end friendships which may have inevitably formed over the years. Becoming a leader in any industry, however, does mean that we have to continually consider our colleagues and the organisation to which we're aligned.

Is it fair on colleagues, our employers, or ourselves, if we hope to remain involved in day to day in-house jokes, camaraderie and conversation, but at the same time be responsible for disciplinary issues? Can we expect to hang out in a social setting without making others feel like they have to moderate their conversation or behaviour? Have we forgotten the need to debrief, away from work, without management or leadership around? If paramedic colleagues are surprised to see us behaving in a particular way, does that suggest that we may not be meeting the expectations or standards we have set for ourselves?

What we can do, with relative ease, is aim for a healthy balance. Attending functions or social gatherings with paramedic colleagues may be acceptable, but knowing when to leave them to it is imperative. Letting our hair down amongst a couple of trusted colleagues, in a private setting, may be the perfect solution to maintaining long term friendships at the same time as protecting the reputation we have worked hard for. Mixing friendly chatter with appropriate work discussions, at every level, is not only encouraged, but it's also necessary if we wish to retain an ability to return to the frontline workforce with our reputation and relationships intact. It must be viewed as a balancing act, however.

Any substantial deviation between being too friendly, or becoming too distant, will cause us to stumble and fall, ruining either our leadership reputation or our chances of returning to the paramedic fold. There are no clear guidelines in this area within most organisations, unless we sign a highly detailed contract, outlining exactly how we agree to behave. The best way for us to assess ourselves on the good, bad or ugly scale, however, is to ask ourselves what we look for in a great leader and align ourselves to those expectations.

INTEGRITY INTACT -V- POORLY PERCEIVED

It's already proven a challenging start to the week, but the hits keep coming. We are out picking up some lunch when our safety team calls to notify us that a paramedic has been injured. The details are unclear, but they are currently being transported urgently to the trauma centre, having severed some fingers due to faulty equipment.

Our stomach lurches uncomfortably, we forget the lunch and head back to the office to try and gain further details. At the forefront of our mind is last week's conversation regarding the frustration and concern that our colleague had called us about. Our sympathetic nervous system kicks into gear, we sweat and feel panicked, as we scramble around looking for information regarding the injured paramedic.

A colleague asks if something is wrong when they see our change in behaviour, but we pull our bluff around us tighter and work hard to regain full composure. All the while, we're desperately hoping that it wasn't this particular piece of equipment responsible for the problem.

As soon as we hear the news that it was a sliding door that caused the damage, we breathe a sigh of relief. At that moment, however, we feel uglier than ever. Our concern had been related to ourselves, the potential backlash or accusations of negligence in forgetting the safety issue raised, and how we may now be perceived, rather than the health of the injured paramedic.

The only tool we are equipped with to build our reputation is integrity. In a leadership role, and more specifically, as an organisational whole, if we state a commitment to action, then fail to follow through, we failed to act with integrity. Our word is all we have to maintain trust and confidence in our role. We learn this early on in dealing with patients and precepting interns when we expect them to believe our word, relying upon this to maintain calm, controlled scenes.

No matter where we operate from within an ambulance service, we must maintain this principle. If we are forced to go back on our word, we can be honest and explain why. Although this may cause inevitable frustration or disappointment, it allows us to maintain our integrity and therefore, trust. Simply forgetting, or even worse, ignoring any commitment we've made, is downright ugly and begins to damage our relationships immediately.

Why It Matters

Paramedics depend upon their ability to size up human behaviour rapidly, with very little information to hand. The pleasant patient who may be hiding intense pain requires us to be skilled at noticing so we can properly assist. A highly stressed patient that fuels a gut feeling that they may want to cause us harm hopes that we won't see their intentions. The kind and caring family member who's abusing the vulnerable person in their care relies on blindsiding us in the hope that we remain oblivious. Good instincts help to form good paramedics; therefore, we must not underestimate our ability to recognise the true intentions of others.

With this in mind, the personal reasons that we may have for choosing to step up into a leadership role often become apparent in our behaviours once we have settled in. If it was about the pay increase, it soon manifests in our tendency to avoid hard work, and our failure to add value to the paramedics in our care. A need to appear superior will become evident through the controlling and unreasonable mannerisms we use in an attempt to exert power over our charges. The fear of being recognised as a bad operator in a frontline capacity is often demonstrated in the rapid ability to lose touch with the paramedic role, as soon as we step out of it. Almost as if we didn't understand it properly in the first place.

Signing up to drive positive change, however, shines through in the leaders that we respect most. How closely they listen, and how their demeanour remains the same, no matter who they're talking to or which position they hold. Their level of accountability and follow up, and their ability to convey genuine care and concern, while maintaining a professional stance that promotes action, rather than emotional involvement. The mutual respect that exists in relationships formed through such qualities and ethics is only achievable through genuine interactions. It cannot be demanded. It will not happen without consistent evidence of the characteristics we admire. It will not occur through false pretenses.

It stands to reason; therefore, that good, bad and ugly paramedics, will form good, bad and ugly leadership teams. From an ambulance service's perspective, attention to behaviour must remain just as crucial at this level, as it is on the frontline.

The unwavering expectation of paramedics is that their focus must be upon the provision of best patient care. Without patients, we have no ambulance service; therefore, this must be the focus of all our endeavours at every level. As a single responder, as a manager, as a leader, and as an organisation, the onus of responsibility falls upon us to provide that same standard of care to all employees, otherwise, how can we possibly expect them to deliver?

Put Yourself In The Picture

If you're in a leadership role, how well aligned are your current work practices in comparison with that which you'd expect from a frontline paramedic representing your organisation? It's very easy, and forgivable, to put ourselves in a different category, simply because we're not working on a face to face basis with patients and other healthcare professionals. Still, it's also important to remember how aligned we must remain. Are you confident that you're leading by example and providing the type of role model that you'd be happy to see every frontline paramedic emulate in the public arena? If not, why?

If you have any inkling that you may be losing touch with the day to day aspect of delivering best patient care, maybe now is an excellent time to imagine yourself in the prehospital care situation. How would you perform? How would your current standards translate in an ambulance callout situation? If you're in a single responder role, picture yourself turning up on the last few calls you've attended and ask yourself whether you're happy with the way you interacted on scene. Did you take over? Did you complicate matters, or were you adding value?

Perhaps you're a middle manager. If so, consider how you view the frontline workforce. Is your goal to facilitate best patient care, through providing the highest level of support possible, to the paramedics fulfilling the organisation's commitments on the frontline? Or do you find their demands annoying, frustrating, overwhelming and a hindrance to your workload? As a senior leader, is your balance adequate between understanding the role and maintaining a healthy distance from which you can remain objective in making decisions? If you still call yourself a paramedic, despite working in a non-operational role currently, have you conducted your leadership practice with such integrity that you can easily step back into line with your paramedic colleagues at any time?

From an ambulance service point of view, is your pyramid structure becoming so top-heavy that more time and resources are spent on anything other than the frontline? Would your organisational approach be described as transparent, consistent and highly communicative? Do staff members view your overall culture as predominantly good, bad or ugly? As important as it may be for paramedics to self-reflect on the approach they take into every facet of the role, this focus remains just as crucial at every level of the organisation.

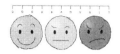

WHICH PARAMEDIC
ARE YOU?

So, let's drop the "we" now, and shift our focus. Which paramedic do you think you are? Where do you sit on the scale of good, through bad, to ugly, in your work practices? Whichever you resonate with most closely today, you must avoid locking yourself in; otherwise, you might begin to lose good habits or could remain stuck in the bad and ugly categories forever.

None of us needs to be judged and labelled, restricting us to one type of practice. We each have the potential to be any or all, at any given time.

If we look at it as a sliding scale, depending on our score, we simply titrate our efforts to reduce the pain we risk causing to ourselves, our patients and our profession. As much as the idea of nothing but good sounds idyllic, setting ourselves up for an expectation of perfection may only lead to disappointment and frustration.

If all three exist side by side, growing our good habits will eventually outnumber the bad and ugly. If we are realistic in understanding that mistakes will be made, a little of both can ride along with the good, serving as the occasional reminder of precisely what we're working to avoid.

Grasping Your Good

While reading, you may have related to every single one of the good points and recognised your endeavours to provide the ultimate in best patient care. If you did, that's something to be incredibly proud of. The question to ask yourself, however, is how you plan to maintain this into the future?

No paramedic is perfect or without fault, every second of every day, otherwise opportunities to improve skills and knowledge would never present themselves. The good paramedic increases their awareness of the positive and negative effects of any action, and inaction, through exposure over time. No good paramedic feels the need to justify their existence by trying to convince the world just how good they are. Their behaviours merely speak for themselves.

The good paramedic continually looks for ways to develop and enhance their expertise. They allow themselves to try out new habits, but quickly recognise the bad, and put an end to them long before they become ugly. The truly good paramedic fully understands their potential to drop the ball at any time. The difference remains, however, in that they continually take measures to avoid it happening, actively.

If this is you, enjoy the fruits of your labour for as long as you continue to exercise good habits. Don't forget to check in with your bad and ugly potential from time to time though, so that you don't lose your way, or get so comfortable in your seat that you forget to grow.

Right now, however, allow yourself to take pride in those high standards you strive for. You may be teased, ridiculed and occasionally obstructed on your journey, unfortunately. Still, you no doubt already know, that sticking to what you believe in feels more rewarding when you lie down to sleep each night.

Banishing Your Bad

You may have begun to realise that you're displaying some bad habits in uniform. Labelling yourself, however, only forces you to become stuck in that role; therefore, it's completely counterproductive and ultimately damaging.

This book does not intend to seek out, brand and ostracise any readers. Instead, it is designed to help paramedics do what we do best. Face up to a confronting situation and work through it with empathy, logic and professionalism. In this instance, it may be particular behaviours that we've adopted.

Perhaps we let our good intentions fall by the wayside due to peer pressure. Maybe we're a little burnt out and have lost some of our passion. Either way, tackling bad habits in the same way we'd tackle a call, provides us with the confidence to adopt our usual tried and tested approach. Every time we catch ourselves behaving in a negative or unprofessional manner, we could treat it just as we'd treat a patient's illness:

- Assess for potential danger to ourselves and others
- Recognise the symptoms and presenting problem rapidly
- Understand the positive and negative effects it may cause
- Gather a full history using every source we can find
- Work through the differential diagnoses available
- Come up with a workable management plan
- Provide immediate attention to prevent further harm
- Reassess and titrate treatment for optimal effect
- Avoid labelling, stigma or judgement around the problem
- Remember how to recognise and deal with it in the future

You may feel uncomfortable or embarrassed thinking about aspects of poor work behaviour that you've demonstrated, but, if you do, this is a good sign! Your discomfort proves that you haven't lost the desire to be a good paramedic, with a passion for best patient care and professionalism.

Use this desire while you still have it. Force yourself to maintain high standards with every patient, no matter the time of day or night. Have a conversation with a trusted colleague about how you feel. You may be surprised to find that they feel the same and are relieved that you've opened up the conversation.

The powerful influence of peers, particularly in a profession where the bluff is so commonly worn, isn't solely a negative phenomenon, it can also create extremely positive change. As an industry group, the less we tolerate any drop in standards between our members initially joining the profession. Wherever we stand today, the less likely it is for those standards to drop. The more we demand, and consistently deliver, high standards of paramedic practice, the more difficult we can make it for the bad, or the ugly, to settle in around us.

Unravelling Your Ugly

You may not recognise yourself in any of the ugly scenarios, but are you completely confident that no-one else would identify you in them either? Self-reflection can seem incredibly difficult when it involves analysing behaviours that we may find questionable about ourselves, and would rather ignore.

Personally, the easiest way that I have found to reflect upon my behaviour objectively is to imagine it captured on video and uploaded to the Internet by a bystander. Should it gain enough attention to become viral, how would I be perceived? Would my family, friends, employers and fellow paramedics be proud? Would I feel proud? Anything less than pride in my conduct is worth addressing immediately. Any reaction that causes me embarrassment, shame or horror is downright ugly, inexcusable and absolutely must not happen again.

It's important to remember that paramedics are human, and, like all other humans, we are susceptible to the impact of human factors. Hunger, thirst, discomfort, exhaustion, boredom, frustration, confusion, fear, stress, physical pain, emotional fatigue, sadness, mental illness, and so many more. All of these factors can creep in, without warning, affect our performance and cause us to make poor decisions. No matter how good, bad or ugly we may ordinarily be, none of us is exempt.

Human nature also causes us to seek out more straightforward ways to get through life and work. Every generation applauds and marvels at the evolving simplification and automation of tasks that innovation and technology provide. As paramedics, we may take the same approach, but if we don't realise the potential for adverse effects, we may not realise the potential for harm. When we take shortcuts, cut corners, rush processes, cease ongoing study, forget how to listen, refuse to self-reflect and avoid change, we may lose sight of why we cared in the first place. This doesn't make us ugly, or beyond repair, but, at the same time, it doesn't excuse the ugly behaviours that we never imagined we'd be capable of when we were first accepted into paramedic training.

If you recognise some of these behaviours in your daily practice, and you're not facing any legal or disciplinary proceedings, thank your lucky stars that you've escaped thus far with your career intact. Accept that it's okay to make mistakes, it's human nature after all, but consider taking action before these behaviours define you. Let yourself finally step down from that stressful tightrope you've been walking between the good, the bad and the ugly, onto safer, more comfortable, solid ground.

Disclaimer - I am a paramedic, with no specialist expertise in psychology or mental wellness whatsoever. If you feel overwhelmed by any aspect of your paramedic role, or the human factors which may affect your life and work, please seek urgent assistance from a professional in this field.

Ultimately, it's never too late to make positive change, especially within a dynamic and adaptable group of fellow humans such as paramedics. Many have fallen into habits that begin to create a negative reputation, but just as many manage to turn things around by merely shifting their priorities.

Why It Matters

As we progress through this book, we may recognise aspects of the good, bad and ugly scenarios for a myriad of reasons.

We may smile fondly at a memory that raises a sense of pride in ourselves or our colleagues.

We may shudder at the recollection of our behaviour on a particular call, from which we learned a valuable lesson in why we must never repeat it.

That's the sole purpose of this book, to provide an overview of the good, the bad and the ugly so that we can casually reflect, free from pressure and without external judgement.

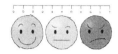

CHECK IN WITH YOUR
PARAMEDIC PRACTICE

Without checking in regularly, we have no benchmark to work from. If we don't reassess our practice overall, we can't proactively manage our performance over time. By assessing our practice at regular intervals, we have the ability to maintain those standards, which once seemed so important, on that very first day in uniform.

We might be surprised to find that we feel great about our individual paramedic practice, but hadn't realised it until we evaluated the situation with the right questions.

Maybe we will be horrified to notice that our standards have dropped since the last check in, but as a result, we provide ourselves with early awareness, and can prevent any bad habits from becoming ugly.

Make some notes at the end of this book to refresh your individual thoughts when reading next time around. Write down a few questions that appeal directly to your own professional standards, to ask yourself now, and in the future, or use the following three suggested questions if they work for you. Consider setting a calendar reminder to review those same questions next year and assess the difference after twelve months have gone by.

Question 1

Remember that every time we see video footage of another paramedic at work, we are drawn to watch closely and picture how we'd perform, given the same circumstance. Imagine exposing our professional reputations to the uninformed and hypercritical scrutiny we see more and more often online.

Would you be proud to watch video footage of yourself at work, in every situation, if it were captured and circulated across social media?

Question 2

The likelihood of us calling an ambulance for ourselves obviously increases with age. Let's put ourselves in an elderly patient's shoes.

If the paramedic tending to your medical emergency, in your future twilight years, behaves just like you, will you feel totally safe, secure and reassured in their care?

Question 3

Our families mean everything, and the thought of them being unwell enough to call an ambulance fills us with dread. Think about the level of care that we desperately hope the attending paramedics will provide to them.

Do your current standards of empathy, care and skill consistently match that which you'd expect from colleagues, if they were attending to your loved ones?

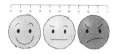

THE LAST WORD ON
WHY IT MATTERS

Every single patient that we attend is someone else's family member. It would seem terribly unfair if we were to provide to others, anything less than the professionalism and care that we expect for our own.

The End

I really appreciate you taking the time to read this book.
Feedback is incredibly valuable, so I would love to hear your
thoughts, whether they're good, bad or even ugly.

Reviews can be posted wherever you obtained this copy or
at

AMAZON | GOODREADS | FACEBOOK | GOOGLE BOOKS

If you haven't written one before and want to know
how to get it done in under ten minutes visit
www.gbuparamedic.com/reviews

For resources, newsletters, articles and more:
Website: www.gbuparamedic.com
Social Media Tag: @gbuparamedic

Thanks for all that you do
in prehospital care.
Be safe, Tammie

Notes For Next Time Around

ABOUT THE AUTHOR

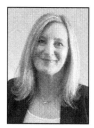Tammie is an Australian author with a passion for professionalism and patient care.

After deciding to become a paramedic, while living in a remote country town, she started as a volunteer, before diving headfirst into the world of paramedic practice. Throughout her academic journey from undergraduate to postgrad qualifications in intensive care paramedicine, and a master's degree in critical care, her enthusiasm has steadily increased, along with the usual study debt and collection of textbooks. Her emergency ambulance and teaching experience includes paramedic, preceptor, trainer, clinical support as a single responder, university lecturer and unit co-ordinator.

For the duration of her career Tammie has been fascinated by recurring cultural chatter around the question of what makes a "good" paramedic. Without professing to know the answer, over a decade's worth of scribbled notes, from countless conversations with medics and students have been gathered together in the shape of this book. Written to provide an effortless ongoing tool for self-reflection in every paramedic with a desire to excel in this rewarding role.

Printed in Great Britain
by Amazon